AR 7.2
5pts.

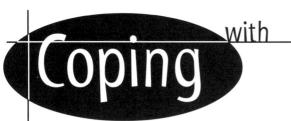

PMS

(PREMENSTRUAL SYNDROME)

Barbara Moe

THE ROSEN PUBLISHING GROUP, INC./NEW YORK

YA
618.172
Moe
1998

Published in 1998 by The Rosen Publishing Group, Inc.
29 East 21st Street, New York, NY 10010

Cover by Christine Innamorato

First Edition

Library of Congress Cataloging-in-Publication Data

Moe, Barbara A.
Coping with PMS / Barbara Moe.
p.   cm.
Includes index.
Summary: Discusses the causes and symptoms of premenstrual syndrome
and what sufferers can do to treat it.
ISBN 0-8239-2716-4
1. Premenstrual syndrome—Juvenile literature. [1. Premenstrual syndrome.] I. Title.
RG165.M638 1998
618.1'72--dc21   97-38630
                                                           CIP
                                                           AC

Manufactured in the United States of America

About the Author

About the Author

Barbara Moe has a Bachelor of Science degree in Nursing from the College of Nursing and Health, University of Cincinnati, and a Master of Science degree in Nursing from Ohio State University. She received a Master of Social Work degree, as well as a certificate in Marriage and Family Therapy, from the University of Denver.

Contents

Introduction

The poster shows a black cat with frazzled fur and a menacing look. She says, "I have PMS and a gun. Any questions?"

A birthday card has a picture of a cake slashed with a hatchet. "Some Special Advice For The Birthday Girl," it says. Inside is the warning: "Never cut your cake during PMS."

How about the story of the bakery with a mean owner. The high school kids in the neighborhood called it "The PMS Bakery."

And finally have your heard this PMS "joke"? A man asks a woman with premenstrual syndrome: "Why does it take four women with PMS an hour to change a lightbulb?"

She clenches her teeth, makes hissing sounds, and replies, "Because it *does*. Okay?"

Legends, stories, and jokes about premenstrual syndrome (PMS) abound. PMS is a combination of physical and emotional symptoms that occur before menstruation begins. If you're a young woman with PMS, you may or may not think it's funny to make light of your condition.

No one knows exactly how widespread PMS is, but most people believe it's very common. Some experts estimate that 90 percent of all women suffer from PMS at one time or another. Others say that as many as 50 percent

1

have it regularly and for at least 10 percent of women PMS is severe enough to disrupt their lives. Some say premenstrual syndrome affects all women, but that some women do not notice it because it's not that severe.

In spite of today's medical technology, scientists have not found a simple cure for PMS. It's not like other illnesses. If you have a sore throat, you go to the doctor and he or she does a throat culture. If the germ streptococcus is the culprit, your doctor will probably prescribe an antibiotic. Twenty-four hours later, you're better.

No simple treatment exists for PMS. What works for one person may not work for another. A good idea may be to experiment with the suggestions in this book and find out what works for you!

Your Female Body

You were in fifth or sixth grade. You were probably in a health education class when you learned that, as a female, you would have your period every month. You wondered: Who me?

Or maybe you learned about your menstrual cycle from a friend, from an older sister, or maybe from your mother. Or maybe menstruation came as a surprise when you found blood on your underwear. "Who needs this?" you asked yourself. Maybe you got scared and thought, "Am I going to bleed to death?"

Sarah had three or four early periods with hardly any bleeding. Then nothing happened for six months. She didn't know what was happening to her body and she was scared to tell anyone about it.

Jan's mother never talked to her daughter about female subjects. She hid her own sanitary napkins on the top shelf of her closet as though she didn't want anyone to know she used such products.

Nancy knew so little about her own anatomy, she worried that if she put a tampon in the wrong way, it might get lost inside her body.

These examples demonstrate that there is a lot to learn about being a woman. Some women are proud of their bodies and know how to take care of them. Others know little about their own bodies and are embarrassed to talk about them. Learning about your body is one way to start appreciating it. Learning about menstruation is the beginning of caring for yourself and your own health needs. It's important to know the anatomical (scientific) terms for your female parts. Then when you go to a doctor, you will be more comfortable talking about your body and you'll know the right questions to ask.

Puberty

Puberty is a time of great change in the functioning and growth of girls' and boys' bodies. The body may begin to sweat more. The skin becomes more oily and acne (pimples, zits) can become a major hassle. Hair appears in the pubic area and a bit later under the arms. Hair on the legs gets coarser and thicker.

Boys' puberty begins a few years later than girls'. During this time, boys' voices change, they shoot up in height, their sexual organs grow, and they become capable of producing sperm, male reproductive cells.

Young women go through puberty between the ages of ten and sixteen although variations can be normal. Breast growth occurs over a period of time, other sexual organs (vagina, uterus, ovaries) grow, and the body assumes a rounder shape. About two years after breast growth begins, you start to have menstrual periods.

Author interviews with young women between the ages of sixteen and eighteen revealed some insights about puberty:

"I had the crazy idea that it was all supposed to happen at once like 'zap' when I woke up one morning. Thank God it didn't."

"At first I didn't want to get boobs because of the teasing."

"I was a little self-conscious about the changes in my body, but everyone else was going through them too, and that helped."

"It felt good, knowing I was becoming a woman."

Puberty leads young women into an exciting time of life. Hormones are the cause for the many changes that occur.

Hormones

Hormones are chemical substances in the bloodstream that regulate actions and changes in the body. In childhood (before puberty) girls have low levels of sex hormones. During puberty and the reproductive years that follow, hormone levels (estrogen and progesterone) are high. Some experts believe that changing hormone levels cause the symptoms of premenstrual syndrome (PMS).

Genes

Genes are the basic building blocks of heredity. They determine most of your physical features as well as some personality traits and whether or not you are predisposed to certain medical conditions, such as premenstrual syndrome. For example if your mother had PMS, it doesn't mean you'll definitely have it, but you may be a more likely candidate for this condition than a person whose mom did not have PMS.

Knowing Your Own Body

More than twenty-five years ago, a group of eleven women wrote *Our Bodies, Ourselves, by and for Women.* Many times updated since it's first publication, this pioneering book came out of the women's movement of the sixties. It may have been one of the first works to suggest the shocking (to some) notion that a woman can and should use a mirror to observe her own sexual organs and the changes that take place during various stages of the menstrual cycle—or during pregnancy when menstruation stops for nine months.

The female sexual organs (sometimes referred to as reproductive organs because of their role in producing a baby) are outside as well as inside the body.

Breasts

Between the ages of ten and twelve, girls' breasts usually begin to grow and assume a rounded shape. During puberty, your breasts grow and eventually when they get to the size your genes intended them to be, they will stop growing. If they grow a lot, you may wish they were smaller. If they don't grow "enough," you may wish they were bigger. Kara observes, "My mother had big boobs, and she was always ashamed of them. She said her mother never told her about puberty. When her breasts started to grow, she wrapped a tight cloth around her chest to get them to stop growing. I would have loved big breasts, but I must have inherited from my father's side. His sisters (my aunts) had big hips and small boobs just like me."

Ashley says, "Not long after I was born, my mother had cancer and had to have one of her breasts removed. When I think about what my mom went through, I'm grateful for what I have."

On the outside of your breasts, the dark saucer-like area in the middle is called the areola. The small raised area in the middle of the areola is the nipple. (Some nipples are indented and some are flat—all variations are normal.) Bumps on the areola of some women's breasts are oil glands that protect the nipple when a woman is nursing. Some women have a few hairs around the areola. That too is normal

Fatty tissue makes up most of the inside of the breast, which is laced with milk-producing glands (mammary glands) with ducts to the nipple. Connective tissue anchors the breasts to the pectoral muscles of the chest wall.

Before we leave the subject of breasts, let's talk about two related topics: breast self-exams and optimal breast health.

Breast Self-Examination (BSE)

Breast self-examination is sometimes called BSE. Although young people rarely get breast cancer, it's important to know how to detect the warning signs as early as possible. If you get in the habit of self-examination during the teen years, you'll be ready to continue this practice when it counts the most.

Do your breast exam at least once a month at the same time each month. It is best to do it after your menstrual period. (Some women get lumpy or swollen breasts before their period; this swelling may be one of the signs of PMS.)

The two main things to do are: look and feel. Get to know your breasts by standing in front of a mirror and examining them closely. Look with your hands at your sides and your arms over your head. Then press your hips with your hands, still keeping a close watch on your breasts.

Check the nipple, areola, and skin of the breast for rough-looking or dimpled areas, sores, swellings, or depressions. If you see something that seems abnormal, such as discharge from the nipple or a crusty appearance around it, watch it for a few days. If symptoms persist, then check it out with a doctor.

Next feel your breasts for any unusual or new lumps. Feeling should be a two-part process. Do one part lying on your back and the other part in the tub or shower with soapy fingers. In the shower, put your right hand behind your head. Use your left hand to feel your right breast. With your fingers pressed tightly together, make small circles on the outside of your breast in a clockwise motion. Go all around, little by little, like the hands of a clock. When you have gone from 12 o'clock back to 12 o'clock, start around again, this time moving closer to the center with each circle until you're circling near the nipple. Repeat this process with the right hand and the left breast.

Next, lying down, again go through the clockwise feeling motions on both breasts. According to the *Mayo Clinic Family Health Book*, seventy-five percent of breast cancers are found either in the upper, outer portion of the breast or under the nipple-areola portion.

What does normal breast tissue feel like? Well, it's lumpy but in a consistent way. The feeling of normal breast tissue can be compared to the way you might imagine small-curd cottage cheese to feel.

Most breast lumps are harmless. One common lump found in breast tissue is a cyst. Cysts are fluid-filled, partly moveable sacs that seem to enlarge from water retention near the end of a period. They often disappear when the period is over. In addition to cysts, some young women have benign (harmless) moveable lumps called fibroadenomas or adenofibromas.

All this may sound complicated, but with practice examining your breasts will become easier. If you have any further questions or doubts about doing the self-examination, you can always ask your doctor. Although people your age rarely get cancer, there are exceptions. That's why if you feel an unusual lump that's not going away, or any other changes that seem abnormal, it's a good idea to see a doctor. Don't worry too much about not doing breast self-examination *right*. The most important thing is to do it!

Optimal Breast Health

Not long ago *Prevention* magazine did a report about healthy breasts. The report said that healthy breasts may have connections to a healthy diet and lifestyle. For example, breast-cancer rates are four to seven times higher in the United States than in Asia. But when Asian women move to the United States, their breast-cancer risk doubles in ten years and eventually reaches U.S. rates. Why?

Perhaps we can link these differences to changes in diet and lifestyle. Diets for healthy breasts have much in common with eating habits that help fight PMS. We will discuss some of these healthy ways of eating in detail later on, but they include plenty of fruits and vegetables, whole-grain products, and olive oil in place of other oils. Decreasing all fats to around 30 percent of daily calories may also help. Some experts believe that giving up smoking and beverages containing caffeine also contributes to breast health.

The Pelvic Organs (Genitals)

The external pelvic organs of both males and females are called genitals. These parts of the female body are sometimes referred to as reproductive organs (important in reproducing and child-bearing) or they may be called gynecological organs. (*Gyne* means woman in Greek and *logos* means study.) If you hold a mirror between your legs, you can see the outer genitals. Vulva is another term for these parts in a woman. The fleshy mound at the top of your legs, covered with hair in grown women, is call the mons or mons pubis. The mons covers the pubic bone; the area in the middle where these bones join is called the pubic symphysis.

Before we go any farther, it's important to note that between their legs, women have three openings to the outside, which from front to back are: the urethra or urinary opening, the vagina, where menstrual blood comes through and through which the baby emerges during birth, and the anus, the opening for waste products from the rectum and intestines to the outside.

Continuing with the outer sexual organs, we find two matching flaps of skin on each side of the vaginal open-

10

ing called the outer lips (labia majora) and, closer to the midline, two matching folds of skin called the inner lips (labia minora). Toward the front of the body at the point where the inner lips meet, we find the clitoris. The clitoris is small, and may be partially hidden by a fold of skin called the clitoral hood.

The vestibule area (the clitoris and its shaft and linking blood vessels, tissues, and ligaments) is a woman's most sensitive area, which is important for two reasons. First, before a menstrual period, this area may feel engorged (full). Second, during intercourse (sexual relations between partners) or in masturbation (self-stimulation), this area gets excited and can lead to orgasm, the sexual feeling sometimes called "climax" or "coming". Not everyone masturbates, but some people believe the release of tension following masturbation helps relieve premenstrual syndrome and the cramps that sometimes accompany menstruation.

One more part of your anatomy you may or may not be able to see with your hand mirror is the hymen, a thin piece of skin that partially covers the vaginal opening. Every young woman's hymen is different. They come in many shapes and sizes. The skin of the hymen can stretch and be broken by different activities. Sometimes it is broken by participating in sports. Other times it is broken the first time a woman has sexual intercourse.

Internal Organs

The inside gynecologic organs are the vagina, uterus, fallopian tubes, and ovaries. If you have used a tampon, you know where your vagina is. Although your mirror will not reveal your inside organs, you can (with a clean finger) feel some of them. The vaginal walls, normally collapsed on themselves like an upside-down, deflated balloon, will stretch to accommodate a tampon, a penis, or even a baby at the time of delivery. Menstrual blood comes from the uterus above and exits through the vagina.

If you reach in far enough as a doctor does when doing a pelvic exam, you might feel a hard bump at the end of the vagina. This bump, which opens into the vagina, is the cervix or lower part of the uterus, also called the womb. The opening of the uterus at the cervix is called the os. The uterus is only about 2.5 inches long and shaped like an upside-down pear. (In someone who's pregnant, the uterus stretches greatly to hold the baby.) It has strong muscles that expand and contract during delivery to push out the baby. The upper part of the uterus is called the fundus.

Extending out from each side of the fundus like small arms with fingers at each end, are the fallopian tubes (also called oviducts or egg ducts.) These tubes lead to the ovaries, which are each approximately the size of an almond; they are held in place by connective tissue four or so inches below your waist. At birth your ovaries contain all of the eggs you will ever have, hundreds of thousands of them. Before an egg ripens once a month, it is called a follicle. Follicles are collections of cells with an immature egg in the middle. Only a few hundred will "ripen" during your lifetime and be released from the surface of one of the ovaries. The ovaries also produce the female hormones, estrogen and progesterone. Knowing about the important work of the ovaries and the uterus in your monthly cycle is important in understanding PMS because the hormones that are produced play a large role in what you feel during your menstrual cycle.

Now that you are more aware of your specialized female parts, it's time to move on to ovulation and menstruation.

Ovulation and Menstruation

Before we talk about PMS, it's a good idea to know exactly what's happening in your body when you get your period.

How Does Menstruation Start?

Sometime during puberty, a gland called the pituitary gland begins to send out special hormones that travel through the bloodstream to your ovaries. Hormones act as messengers that initiate actions, such as growth, elsewhere in your body. One of these hormones, called follicle-stimulating hormone (FSH), goes through your bloodstream to the ovaries. As you learned before, the ovaries contains thousands of reproductive eggs. FSH sends signals to the eggs in the ovaries to produce another hormone called estrogen. Next, the increased amount of estrogen in the bloodstream tells your pituitary gland to slow down its production of FSH, which in turn tells the pituitary to make a second hormone called luteinizing hormone (LH). LH causes *ovulation*—when the ovary releases an egg, which then travels down one of two fallopian tubes. Experts tell us that the ovaries alternate each month in producing a ripe egg.

Muscles in the fallopian tube contract to help the egg move towards the uterus. You may be one of the young

14

women who actually feels ovulation as a cramp in the lower left or lower right side of her abdomen. Just before ovulation, the ovaries release a hormone called progesterone. Progesterone tells your uterus to get ready for the possible arrival of a fertilized egg.

If a sperm from a male has met the egg and fertilized it in the fallopian tube, the fertilized egg will implant itself in the soft, cushy endometrium (inside lining of the uterus). While estrogen causes the lining inside your uterus to grow, progesterone causes the endometrium to produce embryo (growing baby) -nourishing substances, which will allow a fertililzed egg to develop.

If a sperm has not fertilized an egg, the egg falls apart when it enters the uterus and flows out of your body before menstruation. Most of the time you don't even notice it. The production of progesterone then stops and the uterus sheds its lining. This is your menstrual period (menstruation), which in most women lasts from a few days to a week. The production of hormones slows down until your brain tells the pituitary gland to start the process all over again.

Menstrual periods usually start in the middle of puberty and continue, except during pregnancy or in the case of a medical condition, until a woman is in her late forties, although it varies for each female. Then she enters menopause, when a woman stops menstruating because her body doesn't produce enough estrogen to build up the uterus lining.

Your menstrual cycles are never absolutely regular. Using an average length of time, a cycle lasts twenty-eight days, although any cycle from twenty-three to thirty-five days is considered normal. The word, menstruation, comes from menses, the Latin word for month. Ovulation occurs fourteen days before your next period starts.

If you are young and have just started getting your period, you may find that your menstrual cycle is irregular at first. For example, you may have your first period and then not have another one for several months. It is also possible to have several periods without ovulating. This is called an anovulatory period, and it is common in young women.

Menstrual Cycle Summary

You might want to refer to this quick and easy guide to your menstrual cycle to help you understand PMS.

➺The pituitary gland and the ovaries reduce production of hormones to small amounts. This causes the uterus to sheds its lining. The menstrual cycle begins.

➺The pituitary gland increases production of follicle-stimulating hormone (FSH). Estrogen causes the lining of the uterus to thicken. An egg moves to the surface of an ovary.

➺The pituitary slows production of FSH. Luteinizing hormone (LH) is released. LH causes ovulation.

➺Progesterone is produced. If a sperm fertilizes the egg, progesterone causes glands in the endometrium to produce embryo-nourishing substances. If the egg is not fertilized, the production of estrogen and progesterone decreases. Lack of progesterone causes the uterine lining to shed. We are back to the first day of the menstrual cycle.

Your First Period

A group of young women interviewed made these comments about their first periods:

"I was scared because I didn't know what was happening."

"I wanted to get my period. My friends and I thought it would be cool."

"I was in the sixth grade, and we were studying about the monthly cycle in health class. I went home and had mine. At first I was shocked—I guess I didn't think it would happen so soon. But I think it's all about becoming a woman."

"It was just a hassle."

"I was in fifth grade and felt very uncomfortable because I was one of the first of my group of friends to get it."

"It's a part of life—no big deal."

When young women first start having periods, many use pads, which are technically called sanitary napkins. Most pads simply attach to the underwear with an adhesive strip. There are many different types of pads available. They vary according to your needs. In the past, pads to accommodate a heavy flow were bulky and uncomfortable. Now pads are much thinner and work even on the heaviest days. Be glad you're not living in your great grandmother's time. Back then, women used rags (hence the expression "on the rag"), and had to wash these pieces of cloth daily.

Eventually you may decide to try internal protection, or tampons. Most tampons have an applicator that makes the tampon easy to insert and a string that makes it easy to pull out. Tampons take some getting used to, but once you learn how to insert them, you may want to stop wearing pads, or wear them only at night. Many women find tampons more comfortable to wear because they don't feel them. For starters, get the smallest (thinnest) tampon you can find; a junior size might be just right. Tampons come in a variety of sizes. Some tampons are deodorized or scented. It's better to use the unscented kind to prevent any allergic reaction. Once your body adjusts to using tampons, you can start using larger, more absorbent ones, if you need them. A more absorbent tampon can accommodate more blood flow. Some women need a "super" absorbent tampon for the first few days, and then switch to a lower absorbent, "regular" or "junior" tampon.

Remove the outer wrapper. Then read the directions that come in the box. These instructions are very important, so be sure to follow them carefully. If you're worried the tampon won't slip in easily, lubricate it with some K-Y jelly you can buy in the drug store. (Don't use Vaseline or hand lotion; they don't work as well and can irritate or sting.) The toilet seat is a good place to sit while inserting a tampon, because the vaginal walls angle toward the back of your body; they don't go straight up. However, some young women prefer to stand up or lie down when inserting a tampon. It's all a matter of personal preference.

If the tampon is inserted properly, you should not feel it at all. Learning how to insert a tampon can take some time. It can be frustrating especially if you feel unfamiliar with this part of your body. Some women use a mirror to help them the first time. After you get the hang of it, though, you'll be able to do it with ease. It also helps to use tampons that are the correct absorbency. If a tampon is hard to take out when it's time to change it, try a less absorbent tampon.

Frequently changing your tampon (every three or four hours) will help prevent toxic shock syndrome (TSS). TSS is caused by a variation of the germ staphylococcus aureus which in rare cases secretes a potent toxin. Toxic shock syndrome may begin with flu-like symptoms, such as light-headedness, a sudden fever of 102 degrees or more, vomiting or diarrhea, and a rash, especially one on the soles of your feet and the palms of your hands. If you ever have these symptoms and are using a tampon, remove it *immediately*, then call the doctor.

If diagnosed early, TSS can be treated successfully with antibiotics and intravenous fluids. If untreated, TSS can lead to a shock-like condition with low blood pressure; in rare cases it has caused death. If you've ever had a problem with TSS, it's best to avoid tampons completely.

Cramps

Sometimes you might feel discomfort or cramps right before or during the first day or two of your period. This is normal. Using a hot water bottle or taking a hot bath can provide relief. Some women take ibuprofen, which comes in pill form and is available without a prescription in a drug store. A word of caution: Don't take any drug without asking your doctor first. Any drug can be harmful. It's best to get permission from your doctor and follow the instructions on the package.

Some women get severe cramps that don't go away. If this happens, see a doctor as soon as possible. He or she will be able to help you deal with the pain. As we said before, your period will usually last anywhere from three to seven days. Some days, your flow will be heavier than others, but if it's heavy for more than one week, you need to go to the doctor. If you bleed between periods, you should tell the doctor. Overall, understanding what a normal menstrual cycle is like will help you manage your period.

Now that you know all about the normal menstrual cycle, let's see what happens in women who have PMS.

PMS

The study of premenstrual symptoms has a long history, possibly beginning with Hippocrates (460-377 BC), the father of modern medicine. Only recently, however, have researchers taken PMS seriously enough to conduct scientific studies on various treatments.

According to various sources, R.T. Frank in 1931 first used the term *premenstrual tension* to describe symptoms occurring in the luteal phase (just after ovulation) of the menstrual cycle. In 1953, Dr. Katharina Dalton, a pioneer in the treatment of PMS from Great Britain, popularized the term *premenstrual syndrome* and advocated the use of progesterone in its treatment.

What Is PMS?

Premenstrual syndrome is a variety of symptoms (emotional, physical, and behavioral) that consistently happen in a way that is disruptive to normal functioning. It usually occurs a week or ten days before the start of a menstrual period in the luteal phase of the menstrual cycle. In other words, the beginning of a menstrual period usually relieves the symptoms of PMS. One expert put it this way: "If you don't have a couple of weeks free of symptoms after your period starts, you don't have PMS." Some

21

women insist that their premenstrual syndrome continues for one to three days into the period, and some even say they have symptoms until menstruation stops. Other women say they experience PMS all month and their symptoms just get more intense before their period. A few women report having both PMS and dysmenorrhea (painful menstruation).

This book, however, will define PMS as symptoms that occur seven to ten days before your period starts. By our definition, you should have some problem-free, good days after the first day of your period. Also, by this definition, PMS should occur for several cycles, and be severe enough to disrupt your life in some way, such as causing problems with your daily routines and activities.

What Causes It?

Scientists have not found a specific cause for PMS, although most blame a hormonal imbalance. Dr. Roberta Beach, a specialist in adolescent medicine in Denver, Colorado, believes that people with PMS may be more sensitive than others to normal amounts of female hormones. Hormones released during the menstrual cycle may have unpleasant physical and emotional effects, such as breast tenderness and mood swings. In addition to hormonal fluctuations during the menstrual cycle, there are differences in nutrition and brain chemistry. You may be more susceptible to PMS if it runs in your family. In other words, if your mother or grandmother had PMS, you may have a greater chance of having it than someone whose immediate relatives did not have it.

What Cures It?

No one has found a specific cure for this frustrating condition. In the past, because there was no specific cause and no specific cure, some people refused to admit that PMS existed. Even today there are those with doubts about PMS. Those doubters are at one end of a range of beliefs about this condition. At the other end of the range are those who blame everything that goes wrong or any extreme emotional state on PMS. Somewhere in the middle are those who recognize PMS as a cluster of symptoms, each of which need individual treatment. More recently, researchers have begun to take a serious look at the possible causes of PMS and have intensified their efforts to cure it. Although there is no simple cure, there are treatments that provide relief to painful symptoms of PMS. These will be discussed in detail later in the book.

Does Everyone Get PMS?

PMS can occur at almost any time in your life after puberty. If you have it as a teenager, it doesn't mean that you'll always have it. On the other hand, if you don't have PMS as a teen, it doesn't mean that you'll never get it. The majority of teens do not get PMS; but for those who do, the symptoms can be rough. Adolescent girls with PMS may suffer *more* than older women, says Marla Ahlgrimm, founder and president of the Women's Health America Group in Madison, Wisconsin.

Gloria is one of these young women. "When I was in high school, I never knew anyone who missed a day

23

because of PMS. Except me. No one knew what I had—not in my town anyway. People thought I was crazy because I felt bloated like a balloon, my joints ached so bad I could hardly walk, and I had headaches and backaches every single month before my period. Even my family thought I was faking to get sympathy. My brothers especially gave me a hard time. But I wasn't that kind of person. I was never sick otherwise. When I was thirty-four, I had my first child. I had no problems with PMS during pregnancy because I didn't have periods. But after nine months, it started again—worse than ever."

Maybe you're like Gloria, or maybe you have different symptoms. You had a chocolate craving, made chocolate pudding, and ate it all. Now you can't get the zipper on your jeans closed and you blew up at your mom when she said not to worry about a couple extra pounds. You're feeling bloated and irritable so now what do you do?

Do You Really Have PMS?

If you suspect you have PMS, two approaches will help nail down a preliminary diagnosis. We'll call these two steps R & R—recognizing and recording. The first step is to recognize your symptoms or what bothers you.

Recognizing Symptoms

The following list contains the most common PMS symptoms—physical ones on the left and emotional or psychological ones on the right. Many experts say there are as many as 150 premenstrual symptoms. The main thing to

Physical

Acne (pimples and
other skin disorders)
Appetite changes
and/or cravings
Backaches
Bloating (water
retention and swelling
of body tissues,
especially
hands and feet)
Body aches
Breast swelling and
tenderness
Clumsiness
Cold sores
Constipation
Diarrhea
Dizziness
Fatigue or tiredness
Headaches
Increased appetite or thirst
Insomnia (unable to sleep)
Joint pain
Muscle stiffness
Nausea
Shakiness
Sweating
Vomiting
Weight gain

Emotional/ Psychological

Anger
Anxiety
Concentration problems
Crying spells
Depression
Forgetfulness
Hostility
Irritability
Loneliness
Loss of control
Mood swings
Nightmares
Paranoia (the feeling that
someone is out to get you)
Restlessness
Suicidal thoughts
Tension

notice is the pattern of your symptoms; when they occur is more important than what they are. You will not have exactly the same symptoms every month, nor will they last the same amount of time or be of the same intensity. One month you may have mild symptoms; the next month they may be more severe.

The young women interviewed most often mentioned the following symptoms: mood changes and irritability, headaches, backaches, bloating, food cravings, and changes in appetite.

"I don't crave any particular food," said Lorrie, "I just eat all the time."

"Some of the time when I'm having PMS," said Betsy, "I can't eat at all."

Chocolate often pops up as the most highly craved food, followed by "anything salty."

Other foods mentioned by the high school students were:
"Steak."
"Hot dogs with lots of stuff on top."
"Cool drinks and hot foods."
"Pizza and Chinese food."
"Ice cream."
"Pickles, Mexican food, and lasagna."
"Turkey."
"Fruits; drinks with caffeine."
"Cheese."

PMS Is Not All Bad

People tend to think of PMS as a negative state of affairs, but there is an occasional bright moment. Some women report a few positive symptoms, such as increased energy, more creative thoughts than usual, and an increased ability to accomplish various tasks.

Recording: Making Your PMS Chart

Now that you've recognized some possible PMS symptoms, do your "charting." Charting will accomplish several goals. First, it will help you remember your symptoms from one month to the next, even from one year to the next. Second, it will help you and any medical experts you consult to figure out if the symptoms are clustered in the time frame we discussed—before your period, in the luteal phase of your cycle. (If your symptoms do not cluster in the luteal phase, it doesn't mean you don't have PMS; but it may mean you also have a different problem.) Third, charting or record-keeping will help you zero in on which symptoms are troublesome enough to require treatment.

Charting may sound complicated, but it isn't. Just give it a little effort—maybe do it just before you go to bed each night. Try to write something about your thoughts and feelings every day. That way you'll get into the habit of record-keeping. Also, if you write something on the good days, you have a combination of positive and negative thoughts, which will help put things into perspective on those bad days. You can make your chart elaborate if you want to; you can even use illustrations. But you can also keep it as simple as writing everything in a journal. Recognizing when and what your symptoms are will help you stay in control of your life. Nothing is more frustrating than feeling angry or depressed and having no real reason for those feelings. Often it's a relief to say, "I'm not crazy. It's PMS that's making me feel this way." And you'd be surprised to see how easy it is to forget about how PMS can make you feel even if you get it every month.

Becca says, "It was the funniest thing. PMS was driving me crazy. It was such a bother. Every month for a couple of days before my period, I had headaches, backaches, or felt sick to my stomach. I faithfully wrote everything in my journal. A few months ago when I went back and read what I'd written, I realized how happy I was to get my period, and I decided I could put up with PMS because I knew it would end in a few days."

Some people use a page of notebook paper for their chart or keep a notebook for this purpose. You could also use a daily or weekly calendar, or even a diary if you prefer. Or you can make up a chart on your computer if you have one. Make three columns. Head the columns with the first three months of your record. Then, in the left margin make rows for each day of the month up to thirty-one, so your chart looks something like the one on page 29.

Write down the date when each menstrual period begins. Include on your chart any medications you are taking and the dosage (amount). Some healthy professionals suggest writing down the severity (intensity) of your symptoms or rating them with a number: 1=mild, 2=medium, 3=severe. Or, if you prefer, you can write something like this: "bad cramps," or "mild headache."

You do not have to have a certain number of symptoms to have PMS. Some women have more physical symptoms, others have more emotional difficulties. Jill has

My PMS Chart

January	February	March
1.		
2.		
3.		
4.		
5.		
6.		
7.		
8.		
9.		
10.		
11.		
12.		
13.		
14.		
15.		
16.		
17.		
18.		
19.		
20.		
21.		
22.		
23.		
24.		
25.		
26.		
27.		
28.		
29.		
30.		
31.		

some of each. "I crave a lot of sweets. I eat a lot. I experience bloating and lack of energy. My mood goes from top-of-the-world to down-in-the-dumps in a matter of minutes." Some young women have only one PMS symptom that occurs every month. Some have different problems each month. If any of these symptoms describe you, you could ignore it or put up with it as Becca did. Or you may be ready to do something about it.

Allison is a person who decided to do something. She says, "Every month about a week before my period, I got a craving for french fries with gravy. I'm trying to eat healthy foods and I didn't want to give in to my craving. Every month I wrote down how I felt. I realized I couldn't stop thinking about french fries. Finally, I decided to give my body what it wanted. Once I had the fries, I felt satisfied and stopped craving them. It felt good to take control and get some relief. The longer I denied myself, the worse I felt. PMS is hard enough to handle. Why should I beat myself up over an order of french fries?"

What PMS Is Not

PMS is a sneaky series of symptoms, which are sometimes hard to pin down. Those who don't pay attention to the special characteristics and timing of premenstrual syndrome may confuse it with any number of other conditions. Other conditions may have PMS-like symptoms, but there are important differences. Often, our understanding of something as intangible as PMS increases by learning what it is *not*. Here are some different conditions that could be confused with PMS.

30

Dysmenorrhea (Painful Menstruation)

In Greek *dys* means difficult, *men* stands for month, and *rhoia* means flow. So there we have the definition: a difficult monthly flow. Unlike PMS, dysmenorrhea occurs at the beginning of the menstrual period and during it. The most prominent symptom is cramping or pain in the lower abdomen and pelvic area.

Cramps are a part of most women's menstrual cycles. Ten percent, however, suffer from dysmenorrhea, which is a more severe form of cramps and usually starts a year or two after a period begins. The cramps may get worse until a young woman is about twenty years old; then dysmenorrhea tends to lessen. Recent research blames hormones called prostaglandins for causing uterine contractions, as well as backaches, headaches, nausea, and vomiting in some persons.

Although dysmenorrhea is not a serious health hazard, it can be a pain, causing some people to miss school or work. Some of the treatments used for PMS also help dysmenorrhea.

Endometriosis

Endometriosis occurs when pieces of the endometrium (lining of the uterus) break off, escape from the uterus, and become implanted on other organs, such as the ovaries, fallopian tubes, and uterus. The uterine cells mimic the menstrual cycle by thickening and bleeding, but because the cells are attached to other organs, the blood has nowhere to go.

Endometriosis can cause pain, sometimes before a menstrual period and on into the period. The stray cells eventually form blood blisters, scars, and sometimes

31

adhesions (abnormal scar tissue that holds organs together). These scars and adhesions can prevent pregnancy. Experts used to say that endometriosis did not begin until the late twenties or early thirties. Newer studies show that more than half of women with endometriosis experienced symptoms before the age of twenty-five. Most times, endometriosis doesn't need any treatment. But occasionally it progresses and becomes more painful. To properly diagnose it, a doctor will use a laparoscope, a slim instrument inserted into the abdomen. It has a light on the end and allows a doctor to examine your pelvic organs. Birth control pills are used to treat the symptoms. But surgery may be needed if the pills don't work.

Pelvic Inflammatory Disease (PID)
Pelvic inflammatory disease (PID) is an infection that is sometimes but not always the result of sexual activity. If it is the result of sexual activity, it is called a sexually transmitted disease (STD). Originally the term PID described inflammation of the fallopian tubes; now it is used to describe infections of any of the reproductive organs of the pelvis.

In the acute or early phase, the pain of PID can be severe; in the chronic or later phase, the pain may be more like the discomfort of dysmenorrhea or PMS—lower abdominal aches and backaches. In either situation, consult a doctor. An unpleasant-smelling discharge may accompany PID, along with other symptoms, such as chills, fever, and urinary problems. Doctors usually treat PID with antibiotics (often both for the woman and her sexual partner) and pain medications.

Pelvic Pain Syndrome

It's also possible for some women to experience consider-able pelvic pain about seven to ten days before menstru-ation. In addition to pain when sitting or standing, a young woman may feel symptoms similar to PMS, such as insomnia or headaches. If you are experiencing pelvic pain, speak to your doctor about it.

Depression

Although PMS may make you feel depressed, you should have some days after your period starts during which you feel happy (or at least not sad). Melanie felt sad all the time; it didn't seem to matter whether she was hav-ing her period or not. She quit going to school and stayed in bed all day. She refused calls from friends and quit the dance classes she'd taken since third grade. She lost interest in eating, even her favorite granola, and lost twenty pounds.

Depression is an overwhelmingly sad feeling that does not go away—not even when good things happen, not even when a menstrual period starts. Major depression is serious: Nine million Americans suffer from it, and in the most severe cases the possibility of suicide is a concern. The following are common symptoms of depression: loss of interest in formerly pleasurable activities, loss of energy, sleep disorders (sleeping too much or not being able to sleep), difficulty concentrating, feelings of despair and hopelessness, inability to eat or eating too much. If you have some of the these symptoms and they persist, don't excuse the situation as PMS; talk to a parent, a counselor or a doctor right away.

On some days Sally didn't feel sad. Instead she felt almost wild with excitement—to rearrange all the furniture in the house, to exercise, to play piano, and to talk and socialize with her friends. She couldn't sit still. In addition, she couldn't sleep. After that phase, she would "hit bottom," as she called it. She told her family doctor she thought it was PMS, but it didn't take him long to realize that Sally had a bipolar disorder or manic depression, in which bouts of depression alternate with mania (intense activity and euphoria). Most of those with serious depression or manic depression can be helped, usually with medication, psychotherapy (talking to a counselor), or a combination of the two.

Once you've pinpointed your PMS symptoms, the next step is to help yourself relieve the pain and discomfort you are experiencing. Helping yourself can include a combination of lifestyle changes—from diet and exercise, to relaxation techniques and counseling.

Lifestyle Changes

What is lifestyle, and why is it so important in the treatment of PMS? Lifestyle refers to your diet, how much you sleep and relax, and your relationship with yourself and other people. In general, it means how you live. You can make lifestyle changes by and for yourself after some careful thought and a bit of research. Maybe you already have a healthy lifestyle. But you can always pick up a tip or two about becoming more healthy and further improving your chances of beating PMS.

Improving your lifestyle is important for three reasons. First, consider the connections between your mental and physical well-being and PMS. Scientists continue to explore how negative states (stress, worry, anger, and depression) affect the development of premenstrual syndrome. Positive states, such as a sense of peacefulness, a sense of humor, and an optimistic outlook, help fight the effects of PMS.

Second, medical science has not done much more than women themselves in treating premenstrual syndrome. Many doctors believe that the single most important thing in treating PMS is a healthy lifestyle. Simple changes, such as getting more sleep or eating more fruits and vegetables, have worked better than medicine in many cases. Further, a direct link may exist between certain dietary substances, such as caffeine, sugar, and sometimes salt, and the severity of PMS symptoms. One theory has to do with avoiding a quick drop in blood sugar. Some experts believe that a sudden drop releases adrenaline, a hormone that increases blood pressure and stimulates the heart. When adrenaline is released into the bloodstream, the progesterone receptors in the cells can't work right. To keep blood sugar up, eating five or six small meals a day or having frequent snacks seems to help.

Third, when you make lifestyle changes, such as deciding to exercise every day (or every other day), you are taking control of your life, which is an important step in fighting PMS. Making healthful changes will give you a feeling of empowerment, which is a valuable life skill, not just a way to combat PMS . Valerie says, "I used to be a total wimp. My whole identity was wrapped up in what other people thought of me. I did harmful things to myself to fit in with the crowd. Inside I felt awful. Gradually I've learned to make my own decisions. It hasn't stopped PMS. I still have it, but somehow I feel a lot better." Studies have shown that women who take charge of their lives by doing their own problem-solving and handling their anger constructively are more likely than others to do well in fighting PMS.

Casey, an eighteen-year-old with severe PMS several days before each period, decided to try one small lifestyle change. It was difficult (change usually is), but Casey says it was worth the effort. Her friends and family often pointed out her "addiction" to soda. (She drank three or four cans a day.) She denied addiction, saying "I can stop whenever I want," but when she tried to give it up, she couldn't. And yet she felt as if PMS was ruining her life. Ready to try anything, she formed a casual support group of friends and gradually weaned herself off soda. Her next round of PMS symptoms were so mild that she gave up caffeinated sodas for good.

When you make lifestyle changes, some of your friends may not be as supportive as Casey's friends were. They may tease you because your changes feel threatening to them. (They're not making any.) But if you stick to what you're doing, they may end up following your lead. You will find some advice for family and friends at the end of Chapter Six.

Food and Drink: The Spices of Life

Before we discuss specific foods, it's important to acknowledge the role that food plays in our lives. For some of us eating is a way of coping with stress. Frances says, "As a way of treating my PMS, I used to come home after school and put a couple of frozen dinners in the microwave. Then I'd carry my food downstairs to the TV room. I'd stretch out sideways on the futon and shovel that food in, hardly aware of what I was doing. Afterwards, I'd feel sluggish and unhappy, but I'd turn around and do the same thing the next day. Finally, after doing some reading about PMS, I asked my mom not to buy anymore of those dinners. Now I go to the Y after school and work out with a friend. You could say I feel a hundred percent better."

Frances was smart to understand that she was using unhealthy food to handle stress. Most of us take food for granted. But because PMS treatment is linked to healthful eating, it's important to learn some of those healthy habits.

One good idea is to write down everything you eat for three to five days. You can make this list part of your PMS journal. Try to remember how you were feeling when you ate a bag of potato chips and a candybar for dinner. How did you feel afterward?

Part of healthy eating is staying health conscious most of the time. Once in a while if you get a craving, it's okay to indulge. Try not to let your indulgences become an unhealthy pattern. Cravings often go away once they are satisfied anyway. Those who eat healthy learn to do it automatically. If you're trying to start this new pattern and want to know what foods seem to work best for PMS, give your food choices some thought.

We'll start with the foods you eat and the liquids you drink. Let's see what you can take out of your diet and what you can add in. Both will have benefits. You'll find that food doesn't have to be bad for you for it to taste good. And it doesn't have to taste bad in order to be good for you. As you take out certain foods or drinks and put others in, do it one at a time, so you can tell what's working and what is not. Record this information on your PMS chart or in your journal. This way you'll remember how you felt after you ate a certain food. Observe dietary changes all month long, not just when you're "PMS-ing." With today's labeling of foods, it's easy to keep track of harmful ingredients and food additives. Just look on the back of the package to see what's inside the food you're eating. It's important to moderate your intake of salt, sugar, and caffeine to lead a healthy lifestyle.

What To Take Out

Caffeine

Caffeine, a stimulant, increases sleeplessness, anxiety, and tension, which are all parts of the PMS problem. "I can't leave for school until I've had at least three cups of coffee," says Ellen.

"I hate coffee," says Beth. "How can you drink that stuff? But I love hot chocolate. I drink it in the morning—summer and winter."

Caffeine is not an ingredient in most solid foods, except in chocolate candy, however, caffeine turns up in many drinks. Do you *need* it? If you got only four hours of sleep last night, you may believe you *need* a "jolt." Unfortunately caffeine does just that: It picks you up, then lets you down like a leaky helium balloon. Better to take a ten-minute nap or go to bed early. "Jacking" yourself up with caffeine will ultimately disappoint you or make you feel even more tired. Caffeine is also psychologically and physically addictive.

Heather says, "A lot of times when I'm sitting with my girl friends in a restaurant talking, we'll order coffee, or iced tea, or a diet drink of some kind. Then we'll sit, and sit some more, and keep getting refills. I guess that's not helping my PMS."

Heather is right. Coffee, hot chocolate, black tea, and many soft drinks contain caffeine. Often a similar drink without caffeine is available—for example, decaffeinated coffee or soft drinks without caffeine. Remember though that decaffeinated and caffein-free are not the same thing. Even decaffeinated drinks contain *some* caffeine. In very sensitive persons, even a little caffeine may be too much.

If you're used to a lot of caffeine, beware of one possible problem when you "decaffeinate." Caffeine withdrawal sometimes shows up as a headache. "Great," says Tara. "I get rid of one problem and get another." Therefore taper off gradually, eliminating caffeine little by little. Withdrawal symptoms are temporary and should not last more than two weeks. Like other dietary items you take out or add, give the change a chance; several months is not too long to keep trying.

Sugar

It's a good idea to try to remove as much sugar from your diet as possible. Sugar has many different names, including dextrose, fructose, lactose, maltose, and sucrose. If you see more than one of these names listed on a package, the food may contain more sugar than you thought. Other sugary substances, such as corn syrup, maple syrup, honey, molasses, and even sugar substitutes, imitate sugar's effect on the body. Sugar is a simple carbohydrate, that stimulates the pancreas to produce high levels of insulin. Insulin not only makes you hungry but also increases the triglycerides (fats) in your blood and increases the risk of heart disease. Like caffeine, sugar picks you up, then drops you with a plop. Sugar is not easy to eliminate from your diet. It pops up in everything, including condiments like catsup, and sauces like prepared spaghetti sauce. Caffeine, salt, fat, and sugar all "hide" in foods. A good example is cold cereal. Check the label on the side of the box. Is sugar the first listed ingredient? If so, try a different one, perhaps one with wheat as the first ingredient. Ingredients on a package are listed in descending order by weight. If an ingredient such as sugar is listed first or second, beware. It means sugar is a main ingredient. In addition, many juice drinks are mostly sugar. If possible, drink real juice.

Salt
Salt (sodium chloride) holds water in body tissues. In some women with PMS, sodium seems to contribute to bloating and swelling. If you don't have problems with bloating, you need not worry so much. But even health experts consider excess sodium a long-range danger because it can cause high blood pressure, which later in life can cause strokes and other health problems.

"I don't put any salt on my food," says Margaret. "My dad won't let us have a salt shaker on our table."

Margaret's dad has the right idea, but consider that almost everything you eat, except natural (unprepared) foods like fruits and vegetables, have sodium chloride already added. This hidden salt adds up quickly. Through the ages, salt has been used as a preservative. Today we are so used to salt that we don't think food tastes good without it.

Take a walk down the grocery store aisles and check the labeling on a few products. Keep in mind that a normal person's maximum intake of sodium should be 2,400 milligrams per day. A well-known brand of frozen enchilada dinner has 1,790 mg of sodium—75 percent of a person's daily allotment. A serving of a particular brand of low-fat dried soup has 1,340 mg of sodium, or 56 percent of the

41

day's total. One serving of a certain brand of frozen pizza has 910 mg of sodium, or almost 40 percent of the daily limit. It seems unfair—the foods listed may be the very ones your PMS is making you crave.

But there is good news. In place of salt, you can use lemon juice or vinegar on vegetables and salads. Try spices, such as dried onion, garlic powder, or dried peppers on your popcorn. Many people, especially those with heart conditions, must limit their sodium intake. You can take advantage of the many products made for them.

Fat

Nutrition experts say that fat calories should make up about 30 percent of your total food intake each day. Most Americans eat much more fat than that. Too much fat in your diet, and not enough regular exercise, can lead to heart problems.

Where PMS is concerned, however, fat may not be your biggest worry. While you're giving up sugar, caffeine, and salt, you may decide not to worry about other foods that are high in fat. But keep in mind that many high-fat foods, such as bacon, sausage, hot dogs, and hard cheeses, are also high in sodium. Other high-fat foods, such as cakes, cookies, rolls, and doughnuts also contain a lot of sugar. They may taste good but probably won't make you feel so good if you eat too much of them. Cutting down on high-fat foods will help relieve your PMS symptoms, not to mention that you'll have more energy and live longer.

Alcohol

If you're under twenty-one, it's illegal for you to drink

alcohol. But people under twenty-one do sometimes drink alcohol. Samantha says, "When I was a senior in high school, I started drinking a little of my parents' wine to 'take the edge off' my PMS symptoms. Unfortunately I soon found myself drinking more than a little and drinking when I didn't have PMS."

When Samantha used alcohol to try to alleviate her PMS symptoms, she found it made them worse. For one thing, alcoholic drinks contain the sugar you're trying to avoid. Because alcohol is a potentially addictive drug and because women may be more sensitive to its effects before their periods, it is best to avoid alcohol altogether.

Excess Food

In her book *Self-Help for Premenstrual Syndrome*, Carole Harrison, M.D., writes that the diet for PMS is not a weight-loss diet and that neither gaining nor losing weight will help. But if PMS makes you feel heavy, sluggish, and bloated, try eliminating excess food. Eat a little less than you usually do, or consider the old adage to "leave the table a little bit hungry." Try five or six small meals, or a fruit, vegetable, or high-grain snack every two or three hours to keep up your blood sugar.

What to Add

Now that you've removed (or at least limited) some harmful substances from your diet, you're ready to "add in." Adding foods will be a lot more fun than taking them out, so try to concentrate on what you can eat rather than on what you can't eat. This will help you stick with a healthy diet. (You may find the recipes at the end of the book helpful.)

Complex Carbohydrates

Complex carbohydrates include fruits, vegetables, cereals, grains, and legumes (dried beans and peas). You can combine whole grains (cereals and breads) with legumes to provide a complete protein. For starter information on nutritious meatless meals see *Laurel's Kitchen* by Laurel Robertson, Carol Flinders, and Bronwen Godfrey; *Diet for a Small Planet* by Frances Moore Lappe; Jane Brody's cookbooks; and many others that you can probably find in your local library. In contrast to sugar (a simple carbohydrate), complex carbohydrates burn slowly and increase your energy level gradually. Most experts recommend that complex carbohydrates make up between 50 and 70 percent of your daily diet.

Vegetables

"But I don't *like* vegetables," Laura says. Maybe she's thinking of the overcooked, mushy lima beans her mother made her eat, or that tasteless cauliflower, or those bitter brussel sprouts.

Most people today like their veggies raw, or better yet (even more digestible), stir-fried or steamed so they are still nice and crunchy. Some vegetables, such as broccoli, are more digestible when cooked but still bright in color. The less you cook vegetables the more vitamins they retain. Nutritionists recommend that you eat at least three servings of vegetables per day.

In case you're not familiar with many vegetables besides lettuce, celery, carrots, and the others already mentioned, here are a few for you to get to know: artichokes, beets, cabbage, collard greens, corn, cucumbers, eggplant, endive, kale, kohlrabi, leeks, mushrooms, okra, peppers, potatoes, pumpkin, radishes, spinach, turnips, watercress, yams. Don't forget to experiment with different kinds of lettuce; iceberg lettuce contains lots of water but doesn't have as many vitamins as the dark-green, leafy varieties, such as romaine.

Fruits

Most people like fruit. In fact the biggest problem can be eating too much. (Fruit contains sugar. It's natural sugar, but it's still sugar.) One solution may be to limit your consumption to two or three fruits a day, until you see how your body reacts to it.

There are several different types of fruit available, from apples, bananas, and berries to cantaloupe, grapes, kiwis, mangos, pears, papayas, and peaches—and a whole lot more!

Fresh fruits can be very expensive, especially out of season. Everyone says "eat fruit," but few mention how much it costs. Many fruits are available dried, as in apple, cranberry,or banana chips. Remind your parents that fruit is important for the health of the whole family, and if they haven't been keeping it in the house already, they'll be sure to buy it.

Grains

These days, whole grains are in. When your mom was your age, she may not have heard of the nourishing grain couscous, a cracked-wheat product. If she had wanted some, she would have had to find a health-food store. Now you'll find couscous and other whole- grain products in any supermarket. Back then, people also liked their flour and rice white. But recently people learned that factories were taking out the best part, the whole grain. By checking the wrapper, you can tell if bread is 100 percent whole wheat or whole grain. When you bake, use wheat flour instead of white flour. (You may not need as much.) Whole-wheat pasta is available on most grocery shelves.

For breakfast you can make your own nutritious hot cereal from whole grains, such as cracked wheat. It takes only a little longer to use the much more nutritious quick-cooking oatmeal rather than the instant kind. If you have an occasional cookie, try for oatmeal-raisin. Instead of white, use brown rice, bulgur (a kind of cracked wheat), or couscous. Corn is a crossover food because it's a vegetable that is sometimes ground into meal (cornmeal). Popcorn that's popped in just a little oil or in a microwaveable bag makes an excellent snack. Other grains include barley, millet, oats, rye, and triticale (a cross between wheat and rye). Grains appear in cereals, flours, breads, pastas, and as an ingredient in soups.

Legumes (Dried Beans and Peas)
You don't hear much talk about legumes, but dried beans and peas are loaded with protein, B vitamins, and iron. Soybeans, for example, produce the following useful by-products: tofu (solidly curdled soy milk), bean sprouts, soy milk, soy nuts, soy flakes, and soy grits. Other legumes are black beans, black-eyed peas, chickpeas (garbanzos), kidney beans, lentils, lima beans, mung beans, peanuts, pinto beans, split peas, and white beans.

Seeds and Nuts

Nuts are actually the "fruit" of trees. Although nuts contain a lot of fat, doctors and nutritionists point out that they're good for you. Nuts contain mono-and polyunsaturated fats, not the harmful saturated fat found in many fried foods. In addition, nuts give you fiber. An ounce of nuts contains about as much fiber as two slices of wheat bread. Nuts also contain vitamin E, which some research suggests improves heart health and increases brain power. There are many different kinds of seeds and nuts, such as: almonds, Brazil nuts, cashews, chestnuts, filberts or hazelnuts, macadamia nuts, pecans, pine nuts, pistachios, pumpkin and sunflower seeds, and walnuts.

Other Treats You Can Eat

No one has said that to beat PMS you have to live on fruits, vegetables, pasta, grains, and nuts. If you like meat, you can have it once in a while. In moderation, lean meat, such as round steak, pork tenderloin, boneless ham, chicken (skinless) and fish are all excellent choices. Basically, having a varied, balanced diet will keep you healthy.

A Final Word on Food

One last thing: it's important not to get too technical. Otherwise you'll start thinking of yourself as a "case" or a "condition" instead of a person who happens to have PMS. Every so often if you get a yearning for a special treat, let yourself have it. The main thing is for you to make a healthy diet a part of your lifestyle. If you do that and stick with it, you'll feel the results of your efforts.

Exercise

"Exercise? Are you kidding? After a day at school, the last thing I feel like doing is working out!" It is hard to get up in the morning, but morning exercise can make you feel good all day. For some people, getting up every morning at 5:30 to exercise is not very appealing. Instead of setting unrealistic goals, try to incorporate exercise into your daily routine. Whether you do it in the morning or evening, finding the best time for you will help you stick with it. Other ways to keep yourself exercising include doing it with a friend, laying out your exercise clothes the night before, and making it a part of your planned daily routine.

Exercise is hard work, but it is incredibly worthwhile. Fitness experts recommend thirty minutes of aerobic exercise three or four days a week, if possible, but even a brisk 20-minute walk can be effective. Aerobic exercise increases your heart rate and helps your general physical well-being. But even more important, if you suffer from PMS, is that exercise makes you feel good. Rather than taking away energy, it gives you energy. Medical experts say that exercise raises the level of endorphins in the blood. Endorphins are the body's natural painkillers. Think of exercise as a reward rather than a chore. Exercise rids your body of anxiety and tension. Exercise puts you in control.

Stephanie says, "After a jog, I feel euphoric. I love that feeling. The anticipation of that feeling is what gets me up early most days to go running. I can't imagine my life without it. It's one part of my day no one can mess with."

48

Some people need the routine of daily exercise. Like brushing your teeth, exercise becomes a habit or a ritual; you barely have to think about doing it. You just do it. However, if you miss a day, don't get stressed out over it. Missing one or two days here and there won't "undo" your accomplishments.

Carrie says, "I don't think I have PMS, but my friend Ginny did. She was always going on about it. I read somewhere that exercise was supposed to help. So we both got up about forty-five minutes earlier than we used to and started jogging together. It was fun. I felt good and I haven't heard her say much about PMS lately."

A word of caution: Don't try to start your exercise routine when you feel early signs of PMS. Instead start your program the first day you notice PMS waning. Then when you do start, don't overdo it. Give yourself small attainable goals at first. For example, if you choose jogging and do it for forty-five minutes one day, you may not be able to walk the next day, much less exercise. Better to start out with a ten-minute run one day and increase your time to fifteen minutes the next week. Whatever you do, make sure stretching is part of your workout. Stretch before and after you exercise. It helps to relax the body and prevent injury.

"Swimming is my thing," says Jenny. "I'm not sure why. Maybe it's because of the good times I had with my mom when she took me to my beginner lessons. Something about the smell of chlorine on my skin and the relaxed feeling I have when I'm done keeps me going every day. When I'm swimming, I can feel all that PMS anger and tension pouring out of me."

Another idea for making your exercise work for you is to vary your activities and break them up into smaller parts. If the idea of a forty-minute run or swim seems outrageous, try breaking it up into fifteen or twenty-minute segments. For example, you could take the dog for a fifteen-minute walk before school and then jump rope for fifteen minutes before dinner. Basically, any type of movement will make you feel better both mentally and physically.

In case you need help in deciding what might turn you on to exercise, here are some suggestions of the best aerobic exercises:

Aerobics
This category includes aerobic dance and step aerobics, which you can do in a class or by yourself in the privacy of your own home with video tapes or television programs, or with whatever kind of music you like. Just turn up the music and dance!

Biking
Riding a bike outdoors has been an option since the first ones were invented in the early 1800s. In recent years, exercise (stationary) bikes have popped up everywhere—in homes, athletic clubs, recreation centers, and gyms.

Cross-country Skiing
In the past you had to live in the mountains to enjoy this exhilarating activity, and then only in winter. Now with exercise machines, you can "ski" at home or in a gym.

Jogging

For some people, jogging gives a "runner's high" they don't get from anything else. If you live in a warm community, jogging may work for you all year long—if you don't have bad knees. To preserve your knees, try to alternate jogging with another, less-jarring activity.

Jumping Rope and Jumping Jacks

You can alternate these two activities and include a third, trampoline jumping or mini-tramp jumping. Turn on some wild music and get going. Because your jump rope won't take up much room in a suitcase, the first two activities work out well if you're traveling.

Walking

Here's another free exercise you can do every day. As you stroll, listen to music through your headphones or just enjoy nature or your neighborhood. If you prefer indoor walking, you can use a track or a treadmill, or go to the mall.

Anything that gets you moving can improve your mood and change your lifestyle to a more healthful one. Don't forget to record the time, date, and type of exercise in your journal or your PMS chart.

Other Lifestyle Changes

Sleep

Here are two important words about sleep. Do it! Sleep is a great PMS fighter; the trouble is that insomnia and sleep disturbances may be annoying symptoms. Lack of sleep can make you crabby, another PMS symptom. A couple of things that may help: Exercise as early in the day as possible. Don't exercise just before bedtime; instead of making you tired, exercise at this time will probably make you feel wired.

For a restful sleep, take a hot bath, then curl up under the covers with a heating pad (if you need it) and a good book. Try to go to bed at about the same time each night and get up about the same time each morning. If you do take naps, make them short (ten minutes or less). And remember: try not to have caffeine after 3 PM—or better yet, have no caffeine at all.

Some people worry about lack of sleep, and the worrying makes their insomnia worse. Studies have shown that most people don't need as much sleep as they think. In general, young people need more sleep than older people. But seven to nine hours of sleep each night should be enough. You will probably be able to figure out what seems right for you.

If you have insomnia, try spending less time in bed. Loretta used to go to bed every night at 10 PM because everyone else in her family did. During her PMS phase, she spent the first hour tossing and turning and worrying that she wasn't sleeping. These days she writes in her journal until 10:30 or 10:45. Then she listens to some soft music and is usually sound asleep before 11 PM.

Light
Many women say their mood improves when they get outside and experience the healing effects of the sun.

Instead of jumping in the car every time you want to go somewhere, try walking or biking. The exercise will help, and so will the sun. Be sure to use sunscreen with SPF 15 or higher on all exposed areas of the skin. If possible, wear a hat. A word of warning: don't assume that if sunlight helps PMS moods, a tanning salon will work better. High concentration of ultraviolet light is hard on the skin and is a potential cause of skin cancer.

Stress

The word itself with its hissing "s" sounds has a terrible ring. Stress. Believe it or not, stress in your life comes not only from difficult times but from happy experiences as well. To check out the truth of the latter statement, just ask someone who has planned a wedding.

What is stress? The word originated in physics; it refers to the ability to withstand strain. Stress causes your body to pour out adrenaline, a chemical that readies you for "fight or flight." This is a useful response if someone is chasing you down a dark alley or holding you up at the ATM. But the body cannot withstand a permanent strain of this magnitude (fast breathing, sweating, high blood pressure, muscle contraction) for very long. Stress can push you beyond your usual coping abilities. We all have stress in our lives. Too much time on our hands or not enough, pressures of school, job, and family, relationships with self or friends—at times can push us to the breaking point. Add the stress of PMS, and you may feel like you can't take much more.

Felicia, seventeen, says, "My parents are getting a divorce. My mother, who hasn't worked since I was born, just got an 8-to-5 job. I'm co-editor of the school news-paper, and suddenly I'm supposed to come home every day after school and watch my two brothers. They're eight and nine and they know how to push my buttons. My doctor told me that not many teenagers have PMS, but I think I have it. I've noticed there's a couple of days right before my period starts when everything annoys me, and I feel like crying over nothing.

"This one day I was trying so hard to be patient and to hold things together until my mom came home. But my older brother picked a fight with me and I just lost my temper. I felt this rage well up inside me. Before I could do anything about it, I picked up a box of powdered milk, threw it across the kitchen, and hit a window, which broke. Of course I had to pay for it."

Felicia is lucky in two ways. She can talk about her problems, and she has an empathetic parent. Felicia's mother recognized her daughter's stress and decided to do something. She hired one of Felicia's friends to fill in as a baby-sitter on Felicia's PMS days, and she also found a therapist for the whole family.

One of the first things you can do to relieve your stress is to try to figure out the major cause or causes. Keeping your PMS chart should help. Is PMS itself the major stressor? Or is something else, such as Felicia's parents' divorce, the major stressor? There isn't much Felicia can do about the divorce. It may help if she realizes that she isn't the cause, and she can't be the cure. You have no control over many of the events that intrude into your life. You can try and control how you react to some of them.

You can help yourself and your reactions by changing the way you think. Psychologists who prescribe these kinds of changes call them "cognitive therapy." Sometimes call this method is also called "positive thinking."

Dr. David Burns generally receives credit for popularizing "cognitive distortions," or irrational and illogical thinking that can cause stress, low self-esteem, and depression. The following distortions are adapted from a list in *The Wellness Book* by Benson, Stuart, and Associates at the Mind/Body Medical Institute.

1. *"Should" statements.* Constantly telling yourself "I *should* have a healthy diet" or "I should exercise" is a recipe for emotional burnout. Other people don't like to hear you say what they should do, and you don't like to hear other people tell you what you should do. Why force "should" statements on yourself? Instead say, "I choose to eat a healthful diet" or "I want to exercise."

2. *Labeling.* If you make a mistake or an error in judgment, say so. "I made a mistake." Don't say, "I'm a dummy" or "I'm so stupid." (You're not.)

3. *Personalization and blame.* A medication or treatment you're trying for PMS doesn't work. You assume responsibility as if you single-handedly have made your body unresponsive to the new treatment. If you're going to "personalize," it's better to give yourself credit for trying something new.

4. *Magnification.* You turn a negative happening or event into something world shattering. For example you complain that PMS is the worst thing that ever happened to anyone, that you can't stand it, etc. Remember that PMS is *not* a life-threatening condition. Yes it is a "pain," but you can stand it. You already do.

5. *Overgeneralization.* You see one aspect of your life as part of an ongoing pattern of defeat. You have PMS, therefore, your life is ruined. Wrong. Your life is not ruined. You are coping with a troublesome condition as best you can, and you will continue to do so.

6. *Discounting the positive.* Many people are guilty of this one. Someone compliments you on your sweater. You say, "Oh, I've had this thing for years." No! Thank them and let it go at that. As far as PMS is concerned, some young women focus on the negative (the effects of PMS) and forget all the good things going on in their lives.

7. *Emotional reasoning.* You assume that the way you're feeling on a "down" day is evidence of the truth. For example, you feel rather powerless on a PMS day and you say to yourself, "I'm a completely worthless person."

Remember Felicia? She decided that the next time one of her brothers made her angry, she would think in a different way and act differently. First, she would not assume her brothers were deliberately trying to annoy her. If necessary, she would go to her room, shut the door for five or ten minutes, close her eyes and take some deep breaths until she felt calm enough to act rationally. In a similar fashion, you can find out where your stress is coming from and decide to do something about it.

Ways to Reduce Stress

What relieves stress for one person may cause stress for another. Dianna likes to have at least one weekend day in which she does basically nothing. She sleeps until noon, gets up and makes pancakes for breakfast, talks to her friends on the phone, reads, and does homework. In the evening, she watches TV or a movie and has a bowl of popcorn. On some of these days, Dianna doesn't even leave the house, except maybe to get the movie. By the next day she's full of energy and ready to face the world.

Vanessa would feel depressed after a day like Dianna's. She would consider such a day wasteful and get stressed out about it. Vanessa likes to get up early and go for a jog with one of her friends. After that they sometimes bake cookies or ride their bikes to the mall. After lunch on Saturdays, Vanessa does four hours of volunteer work at the local children's hospital. Before getting on the phone to make plans for the evening, Vanessa cleans her room. She knows her mom won't let her go out until she does.

Dianna would feel horrible after a day like Vanessa's. Her stress level would reach unimaginable heights. The two have different ways of dealing with stress.

Since we've already discussed exercise, a few more words may wrap it up. Exercise is without question a stress reliever. What felt awfully annoying yesterday doesn't seem to bother you today after ten minutes of jumping jacks. The only circumstance in which exercise might cause stress is when a person becomes compulsive about doing it. "My daughter got that way about swimming," says Michaela's mother. "If she couldn't have her daily swim, she got irritable. If we were on a family trip, we had to stay at a place with a pool. She exercised too much. It was unhealthy."

Here are some other stress busters that may or may not work for you. Try them for several months, all month, not just during PMS time.

Seek Silence

For most people, constant loud noise is a stressor. Often we have no choice about the noise that assaults us—from the music in the supermarket or coffee shop to street sounds, like horns, motorcycles, buses, and trucks. If you live in the city, try to get away every so often. But a trip to the mountains, the country, or the seashore may not be possible often enough. If you can't get away, find quiet time wherever you are. You may find your quiet time in the morning before everyone else gets up or at night after everyone else is asleep. Finding a quiet, pretty place to go in times of stress can be very helpful.

Find Your Own Place

Everyone needs a place to call her own. If you have your own room, make this area truly yours. Turn your room into a place where you want to hang out, a place that pleases you. Choose colors and a decor that feels restful, relaxing, and stress-relieving. Decorate it with your kind of art and give it your personal touch.

Even if you don't have your own room, you can still find a corner to make "your" place. If you have to share a room, see if you can schedule some private time when only you are allowed in. Or find another place in your home where you can have "peace and quiet."

Deep Breathing

Wherever you are, you can use deep, rhythmic, abdominal breathing. To avoid unnecessary temper fits and angry confrontations, stop and take five deep breaths. When you feel yourself tensing up, stop talking. Stop reacting. Instead, breathe. Concentrate on your breathing. Inhale while you count slowly to three; exhale while you count to three again. Then do the same thing again. And again.

For stress relief and relaxation, you can also do deep breathing lying down. As you breathe in slowly and deeply, you should feel your abdomen rise. Next exhale. Do this deep breathing for at least five or ten minutes every day.

Deep breathing is also a part of many other relaxation techniques, such as progressive muscle relaxation.

Progressive Muscle Relaxation

If music helps you relax, put on some quiet tunes. Get comfortable lying down. Start with a few deep breaths. Then choose any muscles that feel tense. How about your shoulders? Scrunch those shoulder muscles up against your neck and head. Hold this position while you count slowly to fifteen. Then let go of the position and relax those muscles. Keep going with other tense muscles. Next try your fists. Clench them for fifteen seconds; let them relax. If you want to be sure not to miss any muscles, start with your head. Frown for fifteen seconds. Then relax those forehead muscles. Move on to your eyes. Squeeze them shut for fifteen seconds, then let them relax.

Work down your body, tensing and relaxing every muscle you can think of, including those of your toes. You'll be amazed how good you feel when you're finished.

Massage

Massage relaxes muscles and decreases stress. As her first

symptom of PMS, Linda often feels a tightness in her neck muscles. Sometimes she tries to give her own neck a massage, but twisting herself into a pretzel hurts more than it helps. Getting a friend to rub her neck is much nicer. It's not hard to learn massage. You can get a book on massage from the library. Then you and a friend can trade off. If you save your money, you can go to a certified massage therapist for a relaxing treat.

Meditation
The word "meditation" means different things to different people. For some the word means "to think." For others the process involves emptying the mind of all thoughts. (This is not easy to do.) Your practice of deep breathing will help. Sit on a chair and get comfortable. Try concentrating on nothing except your breathing. If a worry intrudes, whisk it out of your mind and go back to concentrating on breathing.

Some meditation involves the use of a mantra, a word your mind repeats over and over. A word such as "comfort" or "wellness," will convey a positive message of healing, or you can pick a meaningless syllable such as "om" or "hum."

If meditation is working for you, you will feel calm and inwardly relaxed after doing it. However, many students say meditation takes much practice to do right. Don't expect too much at first. Stick with one kind of meditation for two or three months before making a judgment.

Marianne took a course in Buddhism at a community college. For six weeks she practiced meditation under the teacher's direction. But she never did settle down enough at home to get into a routine, and she ultimately decided that this method of stress control wouldn't work for her. She learned a lot in the course, though, and was pleased with herself for taking it.

Visualization

Use your deep breathing to start the exercise of visualization. Then close your eyes and use your imagination to create a mental picture. You probably already use visualization without realizing that you are practicing a potentially healing art. For example have you ever imagined a teacher handing back a test and announcing, "Congratulations. You have the highest grade in the class."

You can use visualization to displace some of the stress caused by PMS. If you feel discomfort in your pelvic area, imagine the blood flowing away from your pelvis and being replaced by a calm and relaxed feeling.

Imagine yourself in a bubbly mood. You feel light, hopeful, and energetic. You are in control of whatever problem presents itself. Imagine yourself smiling and people smiling back at you.

Your visualizations are limited only by your imagination, and your imagination knows no limits.

Yoga

The practice of yoga, joining mind and body, is something you can do alone and for yourself once you get the hang of it. But you will probably do best if you start by taking a class. Yoga incorporates stretching, breathing, and meditation for relaxation and healing.

The eastern practice of Hatha yoga, based on physical movements called asanas and breathing exercises (pranayama) is commonly taught in the United States. Dr. Susan Lark's *Premenstrual Syndrome Self-Help Book* has a useful illustrated chapter on yoga for PMS.

Other Eastern practices such as Tai Chi involve rhythmic movements that help fight stress. Taoist and Buddhist monks developed Tai Chi hundreds of years ago as a martial art and a spiritual discipline. Because the movements are slow and meditative, they are suitable for all fitness levels. Among the benefits of Tai Chi are improved circulation, increased balance and flexibility, and internal peace.

Biofeedback

Biofeedback is sometimes used for high levels of stress. It requires training or coaching and involves the use of electronic machinery to help you control physiological responses. This, in turn, helps you to control stress. Electronic devices are connected to the body and the signals are seen on a screen. In this way a person can learn to control internal, "unseen" physical responses, such as heart rate and blood pressure.

Biofeedback takes a long time to learn. It may be a while before you can regulate your responses. You can practice at home without the machines. If you keep practicing, you may be able to cut down on stress, muscle tension, headaches, and insomnia. In addition you will have gained a feeling of control over your physical and emotional health, one of your primary goals in dealing with PMS.

Raising Your Own Self-Esteem

Self-esteem (the ability to hold yourself in high positive regard) is a characteristic that develops over the years, partially as a result of the ways your parents raised you. Although there's no way a person can choose her parents, there are ways you can raise your self-esteem. One way is to step out of the "I'm a bad person" mentality and start thinking of yourself as good and valuable—not because of anything you've done but just because you *are*. The affirmation exercise below is one thing you can do. Then when you start getting down on yourself, take out your list and study it.

Remember: those who brag the most or spend the most time talking about themselves are not necessarily those with the highest level of self-esteem. Natalie has an example. "In my senior year of high school, I started dating this guy named Joe. You know the type—captain of the football team, class president, and really good looking. But the only person he ever talked about was himself. He never seemed to care about how I was feeling. In the middle of the year this new girl came to our school. I'd invited Joe to the Sadie Hawkins Dance, but he broke up with me two days before the dance and went with her, leaving me with a new dress and no date. I look back and ask myself, 'Did he have high self-esteem or low?' I have to say, low. People with high self-esteem are confident but considerate of other people, not just themselves."

Having high self-esteem will help you fight off some of the depression, anxiety, irritability, and other mood changes that often appear with PMS.

63

Affirmations

Affirmations are positive statements you make to yourself about yourself. You can say them or write them. Begin with the words "I am." The use of affirmations will help pull you out of a low period and the negative-thinking mode that sometimes accompanies PMS. Here are a few samples:

—I am a healthy person.

—I am a whole person.

—I am athletic.

—I am artistic.

—I am fun to be around.

—I am competent.

—I am in charge of my own life.

Don't allow negative thoughts to creep in. Just for fun, time yourself. See how many affirmations you can write in five minutes. Then whenever you feel down, read them back to yourself. Or you can read them into a tape recorder and play them back. Better yet, write them on a piece of poster board and hang it over your desk.

Be Assertive

Many people confuse assertiveness with aggressiveness. They are not the same. Aggressiveness has a negative connotation as in causing harm to another person. Gayle talks about a girl she remembers as being aggressive. "She was my age and happened to be my next-door neighbor. The three qualities I remember most about her? She got in your face, she interrupted others when they were talking, and she physically pushed people aside to get to the head of a line."

Assertiveness is different. The dictionary defines an assertion as something stated forcefully. Being assertive allows you to express your feelings while at the same time respecting the rights and feelings of others. As harmless and useful as this sounds, many men (and even other women) do not expect females to be assertive. The negative side of this passivity or nonassertiveness is that you do not get heard. When no one listens to you, you are likely to develop feelings of resentment, anger, and even depression.

Maggie understands the usefulness of being assertive. Her mother took her to a clinic where the physician (a male) addressed all the questions about Maggie to her mother. Maggie politely stated that she could answer the doctor's questions herself, so there was no need for him to ask her mother. As the doctor began directing further questions to Maggie, she could see in his eyes his growing respect for her opinions.

Be Forgiving: Don't Hold A Grudge

How does forgiveness fit with PMS? Forgiveness is important in the same way that expressing your opinions and needs is important. It is important in much the same way as dealing with anger is important. If you don't let feelings of resentment go, they will eat away at you. Have you ever had a cold sore or a crack at the corner of your mouth? The more you irritated it, the worse it got. Only by putting some healing salve on it and leaving it alone did it heal. Forgiveness is like the salve in that it promotes the mental health of the person who does the forgiving.

Remember Natalie who got the boot from her boyfriend Joe? At first Natalie licked her wounds, but the soreness of her hurt feelings only seemed to get worse. She didn't know who to blame, her ex or the new girl.

In her book *Forgiving the Unforgivable: Overcoming the Bitter Legacy of Intimate Wounds*, Beverly Flanigan lists five phases leading to forgiveness.

Phase 1: Naming the Injury This involves figuring out the significance of the act to you. In Natalie's family a cardinal rule was, "Honor your obligations to others." Whether or not her boyfriend wanted to go to the Sadie Hawkins Dance with her was not the point. Natalie believed that because he had accepted her invitation, he should have gone to the dance with her no matter what. He could have broken up with her later.

Phase 2: Claiming the Injury In this phase, Natalie admits that her feelings were hurt. She has no date to the dance and is stuck with a new dress she can't return.

Phase 3: Blaming the Injury The fact is: Joe is to blame for breaking the date. The responsibility is his. The new girl is not responsible.

Phase 4: Balancing the Scales Flanigan says this phase allows the act of forgiveness to begin. Natalie did not cause the pain, but she has pain. If she continues to lick her wounds, she will not be able to move on. If, however, she acknowledges her position of strength as a person with a clear conscience, she will be able to begin to move to a new place of forgiveness.

Phase 5: Choosing to Forgive Realizing that negative feelings will eat away at her, Natalie makes the choice to forgive—for her own good, if for no other reason. The pain that is still there will heal with time.

Keeping a Journal

How many males do you know who keep a journal—one

that they don't have to keep for a class, that is. Edward Robb Ellis did. He kept a daily journal for sixty-eight years, beginning with a bet when he was sixteen. He and a friend agreed to keep journals for a year without missing a day. The friend quit, but Ellis kept going; he published *A Diary of the Century* in 1995. Ellis proves that keeping a journal is not necessarily a female thing. But many women do keep diaries. Recording your thoughts and feelings is a creative act, a stress reliever and a valuable record of your life—even if you do not become America's greatest diarist.

Julia Cameron, author of *The Artist's Way*, believes that keeping a journal is a way to recover a sense of power, abundance, strength, and connection to others.

Laugh a Little, Laugh a Lot!

According to *The Wellness Book,* Dr. Barry Greiff, a psychiatrist, is credited for emphasizing the stress-busting properties of the "five Ls of success." These are <u>learning</u> (throughout your whole life—not just during your school years), <u>laboring</u> (working at something you love and that gives meaning to your life), <u>loving</u> (giving and receiving love), <u>letting go</u> (of the "shoulds" and all the other things that are out of your control), and finally, <u>laughter</u>.

Over the years many experts have attested to the healing power of laughter. Pat O'Brien, MSW, is one of these experts. O'Brien is founder and Director of You Gotta Believe! The Older Child Adoption and Permanency Movement, Inc., a placement agency in Brooklyn, New York, that finds permanent homes for teenagers in foster care. O'Brien urges people to "play, participate, and have phun." Humor is an individual matter, he says, and we all need to get in touch with the special things that make us laugh. He offers a twelve-step approach to "Independent Laughing," a way of getting in touch with your own special brand of humor.

O'Brien gives credit to C.W. Metcalf and Roma Felible (*Lighten Up: Survival Skills for People Under Pressure*) for the idea of a "Joy List." You can keep a list or journal of your life's joys in conjunction with your PMS journal or chart. Keeping a journal of happy times will help you remember that life is good and—most of the time—fun. Here's an entry from Becky's Joy Journal.

"When I was really young, we were on a camping trip in Mexico. It was close to dinner time, and I was starving. I noticed a couple of pieces of cheese on a paper plate. Before anyone could see me, I grabbed a piece and stuffed it in my face. The 'cheese' turned out to be a chunk of yellow soap. When I started foaming at the mouth, everybody started laughing. At the time I felt humiliated. But now when I think back, all the happy memories of my family and our camping trip flood over me, and I laugh too."

In their book *The Laughter Prescription*, Dr. Laurence J. Peter and Bill Dana give many reasons why laughter, even in this age of high technology and scientific break-throughs, is "the best medicine." Some experts believe laughter increases the production of endorphins, the body's natural painkillers. Laughing also draws attention away from pain and it reduces muscle tension. Add to the laughter an ability to see humor in many different situations, and you have a prescription for healing.

Shauna had finally gotten her chance—a date to Homecoming with her crush. Trying her best to be graceful in her new dress and platform shoes, she joined her group for dinner at a fancy restaurant, where they had shrimp as an appetizer. Shauna's family rarely went out to dinner, and she had never eaten shrimp. At the end of the appetizer course, Shauna looked around the table. Everyone else had a pile of shells in front of them. Not Shauna. She had eaten every one. Weeks later, after she had recovered from her embarrassment, Shauna and her family had a few laughs over "the shrimp caper."

In his book *A Laughing Place*, Dr. Christian Hageseth calls experiences such as Becky's and Shauna's bloopers. The telling of these stories is blooper sharing, which is one way of taking yourself lightly and being able to laugh at yourself.

Dr. Hageseth coined the term "gelastolalia," which comes from Greek roots meaning "give voice to your laughter." In other words, if something seems funny to you, laugh. Laugh outloud. You'll find others will laugh with you.

Other Creative Activities

Anything that lifts you out of yourself—or on the other hand, gets you deeply into yourself—can provide relief from the low-down feelings of PMS. These creative activities are as unique as the individuals who do them. What gives you a sense of peace and fulfillment? Writing poetry or short stories? Knitting? Embroidery? Dancing?

Painting? Drawing? Making music? Cooking? Dress designing? Gardening? The possibilities are endless.

Having Faith and Giving Up Control

An earlier suggestion had to do with gaining control of your life as a way of fighting PMS. Now comes the suggestion that you give up control and put your faith in a higher power. For some people, giving up control may be the best way of gaining control. Does this make sense? It's a balancing act.

During her divorce proceedings, Felicia's mother started attending Al-Anon meetings. One of the first things she learned was to "let go and let God." She came home one night and explained the meaning of that sentence to her daughter. Thinking about what her mother had said gave Felicia a new sense of peace. "It's a relief to stop trying to be in charge of everything," she said. She remembered how she'd started her junior year not only working at a fast-food restaurant on weekends, but also co-editing the school newspaper, being satisfied with nothing but As in every subject, and serving as program chairman for the church youth group. "It was too much," says Felicia. "I hate not doing something once I volunteer, but I had to drop the youth group for a while." Remember, you don't have to be Superwoman. Trying to do too much, to be in control of too much, leads only to eventual burnout or physical illness, such as an increase in PMS symptoms. For many, giving up control is part of a strong religious faith, which is another important part of some young women's healing.

70

Prayer

In a recent book, *Prayer Is Good Medicine*, Larry Dossey, M.D., writes that prayer can heal. Dossey explores some of the scientific evidence supporting the ability of prayer to influence health. In fact, he says that prayer can be such a powerful form of healing that physicians should pray for their patients, and family members should pray for each other. Prayer belongs to people of all faiths, he adds, and it can take many different forms.

The Mind-Body and Body-Mind Connection

As you know, PMS is different for each woman who has it. Symptoms of backache, headache, joint discomfort, and muscle stiffness (to name a few) involve pain. Other physical symptoms (diarrhea or constipation, for example) are uncomfortable and can produce a great deal of misery. Finally, emotional symptoms, such as angry outbursts, intense sadness, or crying spells, can influence your bodily reactions. In some situations, the mind influences the body; in others, the body influences the mind and emotions.

In her helpful book, *Managing Pain Before It Manages You*, Margaret Caudill, M.D., writes that your first step in managing pain is to acknowledge that it exists. After you do that, check with yourself to see if you are taking ownership of your discomfort, or if you are blaming others for your pain. Dr. Caudill points out that some women blame their doctors (e.g., "Why can't he or she cure it?"). Others blame family members for not doing anything that helps or for not understanding the situation. Still others blame society for their circumstances, for not making things easier for them.

Becky blamed her parents for her PMS discomfort. Backaches and lower abdominal pain were part of Becky's PMS picture. "The least you could do is let me drive to school when my back is killing me," Becky said.

"Why don't you try walking to school," said her mom. "It's not that far, and the exercise would be good for you."

"Sure, Mom," Becky said. "Sure." To herself she said, "If I don't graduate this year, they'll have themselves to blame."

Becky refused to try her mother's advice (she got a ride to school with a friend or stayed home on the couch) and, as a result, lost a possible symptom-reliever. She nursed angry feelings toward her parents that made her discomfort worse. In addition, by her lack of action, Becky gave control and responsibility for her pain to her parents.

Becky's story has a happy ending. She did graduate from high school and moved on to college. In the middle of her freshman year, she made friends with another young woman who had PMS. Becky's friend Char didn't try to talk Becky into anything. But one day Becky noticed Char's swim suit hanging in her bathroom and asked how often she swam.

"Every day," said Char, "especially when I'm PMS-ing. It helps. Want to come?"

Becky had a flashback to her mom's comments about exercise and almost didn't go. However, rather than saying to herself, "I should go," she said, "I want to go."

Afterward, instead of staying home on the sofa on PMS days, Becky made the extra effort to swim, which relieved much of her discomfort. "Mom was right about exercise," Becky said to herself as she did her laps. "I hate to admit it, but she was right."

All the lifestyle changes described in this chapter are part of the mind-body link that many researchers are exploring today. If you've ever felt as if you might faint when giving an oral book report, if you've broken out in hives before a big test, or gotten a migraine after Christmas shopping, you know firsthand how your emotions can influence your body. In the same way what happens in your body can affect your mind and/or your emotions. For example, if having PMS causes you to give up or "check out," you are letting your body influence your mind. Mind and body are two different entities, but in reality they cannot be separated. Understanding the connection is the first step in dealing with PMS. The more you know, the better you will feel.

Do You Need More Help?

No one knows why one young woman gets PMS and another doesn't. Premenstrual syndrome appears as a complex condition, different in each person. But when you're the one who's hurting, you need more than comforting words.

If all the lifestyle changes you've made seem not to have made enough difference, you may decide to consult a doctor. Even if the doctor's remedies don't work, you will have reassured yourself that you don't have a life-threatening condition or one that will lead to later difficulties.

Linda, a woman now married with two children, tells her story:

"I began having menstrual periods at age ten along with several other girls in my class. Although my mother hadn't warned me about menstruation, she did talk to me after my periods started. I wasn't thrilled about this evidence of growing up but after the initial shock, I handled it okay. In my teenage years, I had heavy periods with cramping.

"I'm pretty sure I have PMS. I don't remember exactly when the symptoms began or if anything in particular triggered them. My discomfort usually starts at mid-cycle but sometimes only three to five days before my period. I get very tired, have muscle and body aches, don't sleep well,

74

and then for a couple of days I feel sick to my stomach and sometimes throw up.

"During college I talked with several doctors about these symptoms. One doctor gave me motion-sickness pills because of the nausea, another suggested sexual intercourse during my periods, and a third prescribed birth control pills. None of these remedies helped. The birth control pills made my periods shorter—three days instead of five.

"Some years later I saw a gynecologist, who prescribed a diuretic. Those pills made me faint several times before I stopped taking them.

About three years ago I talked with my primary-care physician, who suggested checking for gallstones. They discovered nothing. His nurse practitioner was the most help of anyone. She suggested a low-fat diet and ibuprofen, which has helped. I probably take more ibuprofen than I should, and I have trouble sticking to a low-fat diet. Also, the rest of the month when I feel good and full of energy, it's hard to believe how bad I feel when PMS hits."

Linda's story illustrates how individualized PMS is. What worked for her may not work for everyone. And some of the things that didn't help her, may work for someone else. Her story also shows that not all physicians are equally knowledgeable about PMS. For Linda it was a nurse who made a difference.

Choosing a Medical Practitioner

As PMS has become more accepted by the medical community, the need for specialty clinics may have lessened.

In other words, your own doctor may know more about its treatment than doctors did in the past. But you still may be able to find a PMS clinic in your community. Specialized resources are listed at the end of this book.

Some young women have gone to the same doctor since they were babies. If that's your situation, you're lucky. Over the years you and your pediatrician or family physician have probably developed a close relationship.

If you're starting from scratch and don't know any doctors, talk to your friends. See if you can find a physician who specializes in the problems of young women, specifically those with menstrual disorders. If you're in high school, you may have access to a school-based clinic. If you live near a large hospital, you may find a PMS expert at a clinic that specializes in treating adolescent patients.

Your family's health plan may limit your choices. If you have severe PMS or a related condition, your primary care physician may refer you to a gynecologist, a doctor who specializes in treating conditions of the female reproductive system. (Many women see a gynecologist as their only doctor.) You may also see a nurse practitioner, a nurse with extra training in women's health problems, or a certified nurse midwife (CNM). Both of the latter work in cooperation with a physician. More and more doctors are forming teams that may consist of nurse practitioners, nurse midwives, and/or physician assistants, who help with patient education and the prevention of certain health problems.

If you feel more comfortable with a female health provider, request one. Also try to schedule your appointment at the end of your period but before new PMS symptoms begin. That way you'll have a more rational outlook on the problem.

Maybe going to a doctor is something you'd never do on your own. But one day your mother says, "I'm going to pick you up early from school on Thursday. We have an appointment with Dr. Perkins."

"But, Mom..."

When you feel angry, irritable, or depressed, the people around you are affected too. Your mom wants to help you, which in turn will help relieve her concerns. She may worry that something is seriously wrong with you. It's her job as a mother to get the best treatment she can find for you. It's possible she too has PMS. Or maybe she has never had such problems and can't understand why you do. For whatever reason, it's a good idea to talk to your doctor. You can help yourself, and put your mom at ease.

What You Can Do

Be aware of your rights and responsibilities as a patient. One of your responsibilities is to understand that your doctor is not only trying to identify your current problem but also to rule out anything more serious. Although PMS can cause major distress, it is not life-threatening. And although you've come to the doctor because of PMS, your specialist or family doctor will probably do a full physical, not just a pelvic examination.

If you have a close relationship with your mother, you might appreciate her support during the exam. You do have a right, however, to ask your doctor to keep confidential certain parts of your history (such as sexual activity).

77

Part of the physical should be a breast examination. If you tell the doctor that you do regular breast self-exams, she will be impressed. She will check your breasts by observation and feel them for lumps. Although it's unlikely she'll find anything, she is showing you how to do a practice we discussed in Chapter One. All women need to do this regularly for themselves.

The Pelvic Exam

In trying to exclude other conditions, the doctor may decide that a pelvic examination is in order. Your first "pelvic" is one of those initiation rites into womanhood. Candice says, "I thought the start of menstruation was my initiation into womanhood. Now a second one?"

If your doctor is male, a female nurse or other chaperone is also usually present for the exam. The doctor will ask you to lie down on the examining table and put your feet in "stirrups." Although this position may be awkward, uncomfortable, and embarrassing for you at first, it's all in a day's work for the doctor. She can't check your female organs when you're standing up. And remember that your anatomy looks very much like the thousands of others she sees each year. To check the vagina, the cervix, and the uterus, the doctor will insert a speculum to hold the vaginal walls apart. Next she will probably take a scraping from the cervix for a Papanicolau or "Pap" test to screen for cancer or precancerous conditions.

The examination is short and will soon be over. This may be the time for you to use creative visualizations. (Imagine yourself at the seashore or hiking a snow-covered mountain.) Because she can't see the rest of your uterus or your ovaries, the doctor will feel them by inserting two gloved and lubricated fingers into the vagina. Sometimes a final procedure is a rectal exam in which the doctor makes an additional check of the internal reproductive organs with a finger in the rectum and a hand on the abdomen.

Your doctor may want to see the results of any laboratory tests before discussing her findings with you. The tests are unlikely to reveal any pathology (disease), and she may confirm what you thought all along: You have PMS. Once that fact is established, you'll be able to make a plan with your doctor that includes anything you've already tried (that helped) along with treatments she suggests.

If you are sexually active, you should begin yearly pelvic examinations now. If you are not sexually active and your PMS symptoms are mild, you can ask you doctor when you should start seeing a gynecologist.

What the Doctor Wants to Hear from You

At some time during your appointment, be sure the doctor hears what you have to say. Be honest. Your doctor is a smart person with many years of training and experience, but she cannot read your mind or know your feelings about your symptoms unless you tell her. In the treatment of PMS, a patient report is vitally important because of the likelihood that nothing will show up on the physical exam.

Your doctor may want to know whether you are ovulating. This information will be valuable in figuring out whether you have PMS. (If you're not ovulating, you don't have PMS.) You can track ovulation using measurements of basal body temperature. A woman's body temperature rises at ovulation. Before you get up in the morning, record your temperature on your PMS chart.

Be ready to answer these questions: What are your symptoms? When during your menstrual cycle do you have them? How severe are the symptoms? How long do they last? Do they stop when your period starts? What self-help measures have you tried? What has worked and what hasn't worked? Has another doctor ever prescribed treatments such as birth control pills? If so, what kind and what dosage? Do you have any other symptoms that may or may not be part of the PMS picture? Did your mother or your grandmother have PMS? If you suffer from depression, how bad is it? Do other family members get depressed?

Because you know yourself better than anyone else, there is much you can do to help the doctor make a diagnosis. Your journal or PMS chart is important. Be sure to take it with you.

On her October 2 visit, Hannah showed the physician her PMS chart. "On September 17, three days before my period, I broke out in a rash, had a migraine headache, and threw up. This cute guy named Greg had asked me out. But on the day of my great date I felt so bad I couldn't go to school. I stayed in bed feeling horrible. My mom said there was no way I was going out that night. Will he call me again? That was all I could think of. Probably not. Who wants to go out with an invalid?" At the last sentence Hannah started crying. The doctor, sensitive to Hannah's feelings, recognized the impact of PMS on her life. Hannah accepted the doctor's referral to a counselor, who listened to Hannah's feelings about PMS and life in general. She also attended a PMS support group, where hearing the stories of others gave her new coping skills and put her problem in perspective. Six weeks later during her usual PMS time, she went to a movie with Greg.

Possible Treatments

In addition to the remedies you've tried on your own (lowering or eliminating caffeine; limiting salt intake; avoiding alcohol; eating lots of fruits, vegetables, and complex carbohydrates; exercising; reducing stress), your doctor may prescribe some kind of medication. If the prescribed treatment doesn't make sense to you, say so. After all, it's your body.

None of the treatments below help all women, and scientific studies have not shown any one treatment to be better than all others. Nevertheless, some women report that their PMS symptoms respond to one or more of these remedies.

Vitamins and Minerals

If you eat a well-balanced diet and include the PMS-fighting foods mentioned earlier, your body may not need additional vitamins. However, some people need more vitamins or minerals than others. Therefore, some doctors tell their patients to take a multivitamin tablet every day or prescribe a combination vitamin-mineral pill.

B-6 (pyridoxine) is the most commonly prescribed vitamin for PMS. It is one of the complex B vitamins. If the doctor pre-

81

scribes vitamin B-6 in the form of tablets, be absolutely sure not to take a higher dose than prescribed. As with most medications, more is not necessarily better and can be dangerous. In the case of B-6, an overdose can cause serious sensory neuropathy (numbness, weakness, burning, and/or pain) in the hands and feet. Other undesirable side effects are headaches, disturbed sleep, dizziness, and nausea. Taking B-6 with food should also prevent gastric upset.

Some foods high in B-6 are salmon, tuna, shrimp, and chicken. Grains such as whole wheat, buckwheat, rice bran, and rye are good sources of the vitamin B complex. Additional sources are soybeans, navy beans, lima beans, and pinto beans. In other words, if you eat a diet high in complex carbohydrates, you'll be getting lots of multiple B vitamins.

Doctors sometimes prescribe other vitamin supplements, such as vitamin E, or minerals such as zinc, calcium, and magnesium. Be sure to use these supplements under a physician's direction. Too high a dose can be dangerous.

Pain Medication
Medications of various kinds occasionally play a role in the treatment of troubling PMS symptoms. Medications have two names. The first is the generic (scientific) name; the second is the trade (commercial) name.

If headache, backache, or breast soreness are a major part of your symptoms, the doctor may prescribe some type of pain medication. Aspirin and ibuprofen (Advil, Motrin, Nuprin) have antiprostaglandin, anti-inflammatory, and painkilling effects. Many health professionals believe ibuprofen is the most effective simple painkiller for PMS symptoms. You may have to experiment to see what works best for you. Possible side effects of overuse of pain medications include gastric irritation and occasional stomach ulcers. Acetaminophen (Tylenol) is another mild painkiller. Slightly stronger are the nonsteroidal anti-inflammatory drugs (NSAIDs); examples are naproxen (Anaprox or Naprosyn) and mefenamic acid (Ponstel). These medications have an even greater tendency to cause gastric irritation. Tender breasts may also respond to a nonpain medication, bromocriptine or Parlodel. Even though most of these medications are available from a drugstore, without a prescription, consult with your doctor before taking any drug.

Birth Control Pills

Some doctors believe that birth control pills are the first medication to try in treating PMS. Oral contraceptives will do one of three things: nothing, make symptoms worse, or improve comfort level. There is no way to predict who will benefit. If you want to go this route, the best thing is to try oral contraceptives for several months to see what happens.

Progesterone

Progesterone is the most widely discussed and the most controversial treatment for PMS. In the past, some medical experts hoped that various progesterone preparations would turn out to be *the* treatment. Although some women with severe PMS report relief from progesterone, studies don't prove its overall effectiveness.

Diuretics

Diuretics are sometimes called "water pills" because they

reduce swelling and bloating by drawing water from your system. Occasionally people abuse diuretics. They think they will lose weight when they take them. But diuretics can be dangerous because they deplete the body of potassium.

Doctors sometimes prescribe the diuretic, spironolactone (Aldactone), or other diuretics for swelling and bloating, but this drug should never be used in pregnancy. If you are sexually active, you must use birth control without fail before trying this medication.

Antidepressants

Mood changes are rarely severe enough or long-term enough to warrant antidepressant medications. Nevertheless, some doctors prescribe tricyclic antidepressants, such as amitryptyline (Elavil), nortriptalyne (Pamelor), or the newer, selective serotonin reuptake inhibitors (SSRIs), such as paroxetine (Paxil), sertraline (Zoloft), or fluoxetine (Prozac) for relief of the mood fluctuations of PMS.

If depression (low energy, tiredness, too much or too little appetite, irritability, impulsivity) is your main symptom, you should know that women are ten times more likely than men to become depressed. Hormonal changes may account for some of this tendency to depression. According to *The New Our Bodies, Ourselves*, those who experience premenstrual depression are usually concerned with problems that have been there all along. Knowing this may help you ride out your depression until the premenstrual phase passes, or you may decide to get help in the form of counseling or a support group.

"A few days before my period, everything irritates me," says Tanisha. "My older sister Melanie is such a know-it-all. It doesn't matter what I'm studying—English, algebra, history—she knows more and gets better grades. It seems as if I'm listening to chalk screeching across a blackboard. Mom thinks she's so perfect and says maybe I should listen to some of the advice my sister gives me. Every month during this premenstrual time, I manage to get a major family fight going. Afterward I feel guilty and depressed."

Explaining these thoughts to a friend of her mom's gave Tanisha a different perspective on the situation. She decided to ask her family to be sensitive to her moods during her PMS phase. When she felt like starting an argument, Tanisha went for a walk, which made her finally realize that her feelings about Melanie were not all negative. At this point she did not need medication.

Antianxiety Agents

Anxiety can be a vague feeling of dread, or it can appear as difficulty in concentrating, excessive worry, restlessness, shortness of breath, heart palpitations, and panic attacks. Antianxiety medications are seldom necessary for mild to moderate PMS, and they can be addictive. Examples of these drugs are diazepam (Valium), and aprazolam (Xanax). To avoid dependency, some physicians taper down the doses.

Alternative Therapies

Alternative therapies are those not regularly prescribed by medical doctors. Any medication, those prescribed by a doctor or those you try on your own, has the potential to be dangerous if used improperly or to excess.

Here's a guide for evaluating alternative treatments. The list was adapted from a similar list in *The Exceptional Parent* (August 1996).

> ↩ Be careful of treatments said to "cure" a variety of conditions. Beware of any remedy that promises a "quick fix."

> ↩ Avoid any treatment with an outrageous price tag. What scientific evidence is there to back up the claims of those selling the product?

> ↩ Consider the source. Who is trying to "sell" you the treatment? Is it a doctor or other verified medical professional? Is it someone with PMS who has experienced relief or success with the treatment? Will an organization or person benefit from your acceptance of the product? What are the motivations of the person suggesting the remedy?

> ↩ Do you know what is actually in the product you're consuming? Just because it's called "natural" or "herbal" doesn't mean it will benefit you or even be good for you. Some "herbal" products produce allergic reactions and negative side effects.

According to an article in *Newsweek* (May 6, 1996), "Though herbal supplements are no more dangerous than pharmaceutical drugs, they're largely unregulated and can be harmful when misused." Some herbal remedies that are safe when used on the skin, are toxic when swallowed. And some herbs, safe by themselves, are deadly when combined with certain foods or medications.

Acupuncture

Acupuncture is part of the Chinese practice of medicine that involves using fine needles to regulate the flow of energy (called ch'i) in the body and to remove blockages to this energy flow. The application of heat and massage may also be part of the process. Those who advocate acupuncture for PMS consider the condition an imbalance in the body's vital energy.

Acupressure

Acupressure can be a part of acupuncture or can be used alone. Instead of using needles to change the energy flow, the practitioner applies pressure to various body points. Shiatsu is another practice that involves the application of pressure to energy pathways.

Homeopathy

Homeopathic medicine uses natural substances to cure a variety of medical problems. Oil of evening primrose, a commonly prescribed treatment for premenstrual breast soreness, fits into this category of remedies. The evening primrose is a common wildflower of North America. Its oil contains the essential fatty acid, gamma-linolenic acid. Some people say this preparation has helped reduce other PMS symptoms such as emotional problems. If you are interested in trying homeopathy, go to a respected, knowledgeable practitioner rather than trying to treat yourself.

Reflexology

According to this method of healing, pressing on various places on your feet or hands will correct imbalances in various parts of your body. The concept may sound strange to you, but some women swear it brings relief.

Therapeutic Touch

Therapeutic touch is an ancient healing art that has recently been rediscovered. This healing method may sound the strangest of all, but many professionals endorse it. Rather than touching the body as the name implies, the practitioner uses the energy field surrounding the patient to affect bodily changes. Practitioners teach techniques to relieve stress, decrease chronic pain, and increase energy.

A Look at the Big Picture

PMS experts have made the following overall observations about PMS and its treatment.

⇝ PMS is tenacious. You have to be just as strong or stronger as you struggle with it. Linda says, "PMS has taken a terrific toll on me and my family. I feel like I've tried hundreds of different remedies. In spite of that, I've often spent an entire day in bed. My husband's favorite line is, "Why don't you do something about it?' He's an engineer who's used to solving problems. He can't seem to understand that treating PMS isn't as straightfoward. But he's trying his best to be patient and supportive."

⇝ If you are a susceptible person, PMS may never completely disappear. It may go away for a while, only to reappear later. Linda adds, "I never give up hope that one day my PMS will completely disappear. Several months ago for no reason, my periods stopped for a couple of months. Since that time I've still had PMS, but it's much less severe. PMS is something I know I'll have to accept as a part of my life."

⇨ The remedies you try may be more successful one month than in a subsequent month. Linda again: "Over the years I've taken quite a bit of ibuprofen. Sometimes it seems to help a lot; at other times I might as well have eaten some gummy bears instead."

⇨ Remedies that work for your friend may not work for you. It may be frustrating, but try not to let it discourage you from seeking out other remedies. "I had a friend who swore by large doses of vitamins and fish oil," Linda says. "I took vitamins for a while. If anything, they made me feel worse."

⇨ Sharing helps. At work Linda tried to keep quiet about her PMS. But her silence and days of obvious distress made her coworkers nervous. They wanted to help but didn't know what to do. One day Karen talked about her PMS. After this sharing period, Linda told Karen her story. United in their struggle, the two became good friends. The sharing made Linda's discomfort bearable, and her coworkers didn't feel awkward around her anymore.

Medical doctors most often support the lifestyle changes discussed in Chapter Four. In the rare case in which PMS turns a person's life upside down, a doctor may try various medications and offer reassurance that nothing more serious is going on.

Self-Help, Psychotherapy, and Support Groups

We've already discussed lifestyle changes as a form of self-help. But there is more you can do to help yourself.

Dealing with Friends and Family

If you're reading this book, you're already helping yourself get a handle on PMS. And you've learned one thing about the condition: It comes in cycles. Don't assume that the problems and symptoms will go away forever after this cycle. Chances are they'll be back to bug you again. Therefore it's a good idea to talk to your friends and family about it. Don't keep PMS information a secret. One of the ways you can help others is to share what you know.

"I was ashamed of having PMS," says Sondra. "I was afraid my friends and people in my family would make fun of me. But when I started reading about PMS, I discovered that I had information other people were interested in hearing. For example, this is what happened to me when I moved into my first apartment.

"It was the summer after high school. I wasn't ready for college, but I didn't want to live at home anymore. I got a chance to share a house with two other girls. I wondered if it would work out, but they seemed nice.

"The day I moved in, Collette, the businesslike one, acted sort of disinterested. Rhonda, the one I knew better, acted bossy. I was practically in tears, thinking I'd made a huge mistake.

"Two days later I found out that they'd both just gotten their periods. They were like different people. Rhonda apologized for the way she'd acted. Then I told both of them something I'd just read. People who live in the same place often get their periods at the same time. So that meant there might soon be three of us 'PMS-ing' together. We all had a good laugh, which really cleared the air."

For Sondra, Collette, and Rhonda, this information brought the group closer together. Right away, they started putting up imaginary "red flags" on PMS days. The three of them vowed to try to be more considerate, supportive, and forgiving of each other during these times. If you're still living at home, you may need to point out to brothers, sisters, and your parents what a nice person you are to live with most of the time. Ask if they'll cut you some slack during PMS time.

Planning Around PMS

If physical discomfort and mood problems affect you premenstrually, you may find advance planning helpful. PMS comes around every month with annoying regularity. Why not plan for it? Here are a few things you can do:

☞Schedule fewer activities (perhaps only the necessary ones) on the days you suspect symptoms will be most severe. Make yourself less busy, and plan to devote more time to pampering yourself or doing whatever you need to do to gain control. A bubble bath? Exercise? Spending more time alone? Listening to your favorite tunes?

↪ In order to do less on PMS days, you may have to accomplish more during the rest of your cycle.

↪ Figure out what you will want or need on PMS days. Tell your family about your plan to post a list somewhere, such as on the refrigerator, for all to see. Here is Celeste's list. "Today I would like to: 1) Go with Lonnie to work out at the Y. 2) Make my own dinner when I get home. 3) Do my job (dishes) when I'm done with dinner. 4) Do my homework after that." Celeste's family (her younger sister, two older brothers, her mother and father) took to this list-posting with ease. Now they knew exactly what to expect.

Accept Support

The advice to accept support may seem unnecessary at best and silly at worst, but it can't hurt you to hear it anyway. It's not someone else's responsibility to remember to give you support. You may have to ask. Even though PMS may feel just as bad, it is not something that shows like an infected finger or a broken leg.

As strange as it seems, you may have fallen into the habit of going it alone. Says Stephanie, "People just don't understand. How could they? Especially my boyfriend. He doesn't have PMS."

What Stephanie says is true. Only you can feel what you're feeling. But people who love you do want to help. They probably don't know what to do. You may need to tell them.

"But I don't know what to tell them," Stephanie says. "How can they understand when I don't know myself?"

What Stephanie needs to say, though it won't be easy, is that she doesn't know exactly what she needs. She may have to tell her boyfriend that she values his support and expressions of caring, and that during her PMS she needs him to show her these even more.

Dealing with Anger and Depression

Managing anger is a job for everyone, not just for those with PMS. Everyone gets mad; some people feel angry several times a day. Others carry their anger around like a purse full of stones. Someone who says, "I never get angry," maybe ignoring her feelings and may have trouble recognizing her own anger.

Anger is not a bad emotion. In fact, anger can be very useful. Feelings of outrage are often catalysts for accomplishing important tasks. For example, anger at overflowing landfills fueled the recycling effort. Anger over the unjust treatment of African Americans started the civil rights movement.

Turning anger inward and causing depression is unhealthy, but so is letting it explode. In *The Dance of Anger: A Woman's Guide to Changing the Patterns of Intimate Relationships*, Harriet Goldhor Lerner says that venting our anger does no good unless we also change our unhealthy ways of relating to others. She identifies two common patterns in women: the "nice-lady" category and the "bitch" category. Both reinforce old patterns and keep change from happening. "Nice ladies" are afraid to express anger even when an expression of true feelings is justified. These women's anger eventually explodes at inappropriate times, and they end up feeling guilty. A "bitchy" woman may spend her energy trying (unsuccessfully) to change another person instead of focusing on herself. Both ways of relating make women feel powerless and lead to further anger.

Psychologist Susan Heitler (in the *Rocky Mountain News*, October 23, 1996) said that people who are depressed have aimed their anger inward and usually feel mad at themselves. They are actually mad at someone (something) that has taken away their control. If we apply this theory to PMS, it's no wonder that people become furious and depressed over a condition that seems to have a will of its own. Obviously, the only way to conquer PMS is to gain control over it.

If you lose it, by having a temper tantrum or going into a rage, what's in control? Your anger is. And you're not.

The Institute for Mental Health Initiatives suggests that when you start to get angry, you consider one word: RETHINK.

R stands for *recognize*. Recognize and acknowledge your anger.

E stands for *empathize*. The dictionary defines empathy as "understanding so intimate that the feelings, thoughts, and motives of one are readily comprehended by another." In other words, trying to understand where another person is coming from. This can be a hard step when you're steaming mad, but give it a try.

Think about the anger-producing incident in a new and different way. Can you see humor in the situation? Did you have a part in the problem? Do you have any ideas for solving it?

Hear what the other person has to say. Really listen. Repeat back what you think you heard.

Integrate love and/or respect. Use "I" messages to state your opinion on how what happened makes you feel. "I" messages are statements about how *you* feel as opposed to statements condemning another's behavior. For example, "I feel discounted when someone doesn't listen to me." Another: "I feel angry when I am interrupted."

Notice what works in controlling your anger. Exercise, journal keeping, hot baths, hugs?

Keep your focus on the present. Don't rehash old hurts or bring up grudges.

Let's see how the RETHINK method might play out in actual practice.

The Scene: You're definitely in your PMS phase. Your hands and feet are swollen, your head is pounding, and your lower abdominal area feels like it's been punched. As a way of gaining control, you decide to wear your favorite blouse, the one you ironed two days ago. You look for it in the closet; it's not there.

Of course, your sister has it. She always borrows your clothes without asking. But she knows it's your favorite blouse, and she saw you ironing it. How could she? You want to strangle her, but she's already gone to school. What can you do? You'd like to rip her clothes to shreds.

But wait. You've written RETHINK across your bedroom mirror. You're ready to try this new method.

Recognize your anger? No problem with that. You're furious!

Empathize? See the situation from her viewpoint? Well, you have borrowed her clothes at times.

Think about the situation in a new way. Maybe you could get her to loan you her new dress for your date this weekend.

Listen to her. She isn't here now, but you'll see her at school. She'd better have a good reason.

Integrate respect and love. You do love her. You've had a lot of fun times together. And she is your only sister.

Notice what works to control your anger. It would probably help to write her a note. It always makes you feel better to express your feelings in writing.

Keep your attention on the present. You have to. You don't have time to bring up all the other times your sister has borrowed your clothes. You have more important things to do.

If Rethink is too hard to remember, here's something easier to use when you get angry:

When you feel angry, think of a traffic light: red, yellow, and green.

Red: Stop. Don't react. Isolate yourself, if necessary.

Yellow: Take some time, maybe until the end of your PMS phase.

Green: Find the person with whom you've disagreed. Talk things over.

Helpers: Counselors and Therapists

If you have severe mood swings or depression or if you

feel you cannot relieve your stress alone, you may decide to talk with a counselor.

Margot believed that her feelings of low self-worth and her once-a-month blowups at friends and family were interfering with her relationships. She wanted to see a counselor. But where would she find one? Thanks to a friend's suggestion, she had her first visit four months ago with Lynn, a licensed clinical social worker. Lynn's office is a couple of miles from Margot's house. Margot rides her bike to her appointments. At first Lynn simply provided a listening ear, with no interruptions or corrections. After five visits, Lynn suggested that Margot might want to get an evaluation for antidepressant medication.

Margot agreed and had one visit with Dr. Wiseman, a male psychiatrist. After going over the possible benefits and side effects of the medication with Margot and her mother, Dr. Wiseman prescribed a low daily dose of Prozac, which Margot took for two months. At the end of this time, Margot decided that her weekly visits with Lynn had made her feel much better. Under Dr. Wiseman's direction, she discontinued the use of Prozac and contin-ued her weekly sessions with Lynn.

You don't have to have a major mood disorder to ben-efit from seeing a counselor. Almost everyone can use this kind of support from time to time. Sometimes because of attitudes within their families, young women feel ashamed or embarrassed to take this step ("I'm not crazy. Why should I see a therapist?") Look at it this way: If you had strep throat, would you refuse to take penicillin? If you had an infected toe, would you avoid medical treat-ment?

Because there are so many types of helpers with so many different attitudes and abilities, you can't be too careful in choosing one. Depending on where you live, your mode of transportation, your health insurance, and your finances, you may not have much choice. However, you always have the choice to stop therapy if the therapist you've chosen is not helpful.

States differ in the ways they regulate mental health professionals. Therapist, counselor, and psychotherapist are generic terms that anyone can use. People who put these titles after their names may or may not be certified or licensed in your state.

A certified therapist has completed specialized training and should have a certificate to prove it. Angie's mother had a master's degree in nursing and for many years taught at the college level. She attended a part-time program in family therapy for two years and received her certificate. Although she is now a certified therapist, she would need to spend many more hours in supervised practice in order to become a licensed marriage and family therapist.

A licensed therapist, such as a licensed clinical social worker, has met various requirements for practicing in the state and has passed an examination by the state board of examiners. This person may use initials, such as LCSW for licensed clinical social worker, after his or her name.

Usually, professionals such as psychiatrists, psychiatric nurses, psychologists, and social workers are regulated by a state board. If you have questions about a therapist's license or other general questions about qualifications, ask the therapist or call the appropriate state board. You should be able to find a listing in the telephone directory.

Just as you have rights as a consumer of medical services, you have rights as a consumer of mental health services. It's extremely important to feel comfortable with a mental health worker. The National Organization for Women (NOW) has developed a Bill of Rights for the consumer of psychotherapy. The questions below are adapted from it.

Your first right, which is the foundation for all the rest, is the right to ask questions, such as:

1. How do you feel about women and their special circumstances?

2. What is your training, what are your qualifications, how long have you done this work, and how much experience have you had with emotional problems related to PMS?

3. What are your appointment policies and procedures? (For example, many mental health professionals charge for an appointment that is not canceled twenty-four hours in advance.)

4. What are your fees, and where does my health insurance fit in?

5. Is what I say to you confidential?

6. What is your policy regarding the termination of therapy?

Most mental health practitioners disclose this type of information on the first visit. Some offer you an informational visit without charge.

Types of Mental Health Professionals

☞ Counselors are most often priests, ministers, or

laypersons from a particular religious tradition. They are sometimes called pastoral counselors.

⇝ Those with an undergraduate degree in social work can put the initials BSW after their names. They may be called social workers. Those with a master's degree in social work use the initials MSW. If they have had a required number of supervised hours in a clinical setting and have passed the state licensing exam, they can use the initials LCSW (or similar initials).

⇝ Although some people call themselves "psychologists" with just a master's degree, clinical psychologists should have a doctorate (Ph.D.), have a large number of supervised hours of practice, and be licensed in their state. Although Ph.D. psychologists may have trained in the medical tradition, they are not medical doctors and cannot prescribe medications.

⇝ Psychiatrists are medical doctors with specialized training in psychiatry, the science of mental disorders. A psychiatrist has had four years of medical school training after college plus several years of specialized training in psychiatry. A psychiatrist may be the specialist who prescribes and monitors medications for anxiety and depression. You may have a psychiatrist as your primary mental-health counselor, or she may be an occasional consultant. Fees for psychiatrists are usually higher than those for other therapists.

⇝ Family therapists may have their basic training in

pastoral counseling, social work, psychology, or psychiatry. They have then taken further training in dealing with a person as a member of a family group. In therapy, they often bring in other family members and emphasize the influence of the family (perhaps for many past generations) on the client.

When you are choosing a therapist, the main thing to evaluate is how that person works with you. Are you comfortable with the person? Do you feel better after your sessions? (Sometimes people don't feel "good" after a session but believe they have made progress in problem-solving or working on difficult issues in their lives.)

Support Groups

Informal Support Groups

Support groups don't have to be large; you and one other person can make up a group of two. In fact, the person most often mentioned as a support by the young women interviewed was Mom. Mom's help ranged from explaining about menstruation to giving advice on pain medications.

"I was excited to get my first period. I told my mom, and she took me out to dinner to celebrate my womanhood."

"My mother gave me information about my heredity, as well as some ideas for solutions to my problems caused by PMS."

"My mom got me a heating pad and sometimes makes me a cup of herbal tea."

"My mom took me to the doctor. He gave me birth control pills, which helped."

"My mother reassured me that everything was okay."
"She listens to me."
Young women also mentioned female friends as supports.
"My best friend Monica and I watch sad movies together when one of us is PMS-ing. We've become closer because of what we've gone through together."
"Sally and I give each other comfort and help each other out in any way we can."
"At PMS time my friends know where I'm coming from. They know when to push and when to back off."
Some young women identified a male friend as a support. Here is one example.
"My boyfriend is great when I'm having PMS. He rubs my back or my tummy and makes me feel good about myself."

Formal Support Groups

A formal support group may be hard to find. If you live in a big city, you may be able to locate one through a university medical center or PMS clinic. If you are seeing a physician or alternative medical person, be sure to ask for a referral to a group. A support group may be a supplement to medical treatment or may be a person's main resource for help. Sometimes in the absence of a PMS group, young women find support at a 12-step program, such as Al-Anon or Overeaters Anonymous. The problem isn't the same, but the coping mechanisms may be similar. (And be sure to check the resources listed at the end of this book.)

If you can't find a support group, you may want to start one yourself. If you can get two or three people together on a regular basis, you have your group. Be sure to keep the discussion upbeat, focusing on remedies that have helped.

If you find someone to talk to on the Internet, be sure to remember that what you are learning may be only one person's opinion and not a treatment that has been scientifically tested.

Finally, try reading some of the latest reports on research into the causes and treatment of PMS. These days scientists are not only taking premenstrual syndrome seriously but are testing new and better ways of treating it.

Advice for Family and Friends

If you're a family member or a friend of a young woman with PMS, you have probably felt as helpless as the person with the symptoms. Maybe you've felt even more helpless. At least the affected person can do something— exercise, make dietary changes, get more sleep, see a therapist. What can you do?

The most important thing for you to do is "be there." A person with PMS can feel alone and emotionally isolated.

Start by being a listener. For most of us, active listening is a hard job. We want to do the talking. But during PMS time for your daughter, sister, or friend, try to tune in to her words and her feelings. Open-ended comments such as, "I bet you get tired of going through this every month" may elicit a "yes," more feelings, and the comment that you are very understanding. Sometimes your friend doesn't want advice; she just wants to talk.

Here is a conversation between Holly, a young woman with PMS, and her friend, Natasha.

Holly: "I hate Miss Sneedgrass. For some reason she doesn't like me. I should have had an A on that paper instead of a C+."

Natasha: "It almost seems as if Miss S has it in for you."

Holly: "It sure does. And Rachel can do no wrong. Miss S just pretends she doesn't hear when Rachel whispers all through class. But let me close my eyes for a second, and she's knocking on my desk. I couldn't sleep last night; I had my usual PMS nightmares."

Natasha: "You could have stayed home from school today, but there you were."

Holly: "Darned right! Rachel skips class more often than she comes, but nobody notices."

Natasha: "It feels crummy when you're trying hard, and people don't seem to care."

Holly: "You know what, Natasha. You're a great friend. How was your day?"

In the exchange, Natasha simply mirrored Holly's emotions. As a result, Holly felt understood, and Natasha felt as if she had actually done something to improve her friend's mood.

Second, in addition to offering a listening ear, you can provide a sense of connection by touch. In other words, get physical. Show your love and concern with a light touch on the arm. A hug or a kiss often speaks louder than hundreds of words.

Third, get her outside. She may need some time alone; honor that request. But too much time inside can lead to a feeling of isolation. See if she'll go for a walk with you. Or you could offer to help her with some of her work, so she could go for a walk alone.

Fourth, don't take personally your friend's angry outbursts. Before you respond, wait for your anger to subside. While you're waiting, see if you can figure out where she's coming from. See if you can understand the reason behind the emotion. If her anger seems irrational to you, say something like: "I know you think I don't understand, and maybe I don't, but I'm trying." Then let go of any guilt you have. You did your best.

Fifth, bring her some food. How about a bowl of air-popped popcorn or some fruit. Be sure to show some knowledge of the dietary changes she's trying to make. How about bringing her a cup of herbal tea on a tray with some flowers?

Sixth, don't attempt to control her life. What she does about PMS is her business. Of course, you can make suggestions if she wants them. You can cut out newspaper and magazine articles and you can go with her to medical appointments or a support group. But let her tell you what she wants to do about PMS. Any other approach is unlikely to work.

Mandy's mother was always dragging her to the doctor or offering pain pills that Mandy didn't want. The result was an angry, irritable daughter and a frustrated mother. Don't expect to be able to cure your daughter's PMS. It's her PMS, and she deserves the chance to attack it in her own way. Letting her take control is an important part of the healing process.

In Chapter 7 you'll get an idea of some foods that help fight PMS. You'll find recipes in each of five food groups.

Healthy Recipes for the Busy Young Woman

Because healthful eating is such an important part of PMS control, let's talk about a lifelong plan.

Proteins, Carbohydrates, and Fats

Nutritionists divide foods into these categories: proteins, carbohydrates, fats, vitamins, and minerals.

Proteins, made up of smaller units called amino acids, are important in the making of hormones, muscle tissue, and enzymes.

Carbohydrates are either simple or complex. Sugar is a simple carbohydrate. Complex carbohydrates are made up of chains of sugars. A generation ago, people thought that eating complex carbohydrates, such as potatoes and pasta, would make them overweight. Experts now understand that this is not true and advise the consumption of more complex carbohydrates.

Fats are classified as saturated or unsaturated. Experts advise avoiding an overload of all fats but especially of saturated. These are the ones that make people more prone to heart disease. The nutrition labels on all packaged foods will tell you how much saturated and nonsaturated fat are in the food products.

Vitamins and *minerals* assist with various body func-
tions and occur naturally in the food groups recommend-
ed below. Other than a daily multivitamin, which some
doctors suggest, vitamin supplements may not be necessary
and can be dangerous in large doses.

The U.S. Department of Agriculture and the U.S.
Department of Health and Human Services regularly
publish *Dietary Guidelines for Americans* to help you
make responsible food choices. The Food Guide
Pyramid, which you may have seen on your bread wrap-
pers or cereal boxes, includes five major food groups
that serve as the basis for everyday good eating. The
largest sections (the ones nearest the bottom of the pyramid) include foods we need to eat the most. These foods
come from plants.

↝ At the bottom of the pyramid is the Grain Products
Group. This group includes cold cereals, hot cereals, bread, rice, noodles, and grains. Choose nine
to eleven servings a day from this group.

↝ Sharing the next level of the pyramid are the
Vegetable Group (three to five servings) and the
Fruit Group (two to four servings a day).

↝ Next comes the Dairy Group (milk, yogurt, and
cheese). Adults do well with two to three servings
a day from this group, but young people between
the ages of eleven and twenty-four should have
five servings per day. During adolescence, the
bones grow fast and have an increased need for the
calcium in the Dairy Group and in some fortified
foods. On the same level is the Meat and Beans

Group (lean meat, poultry, fish, dry beans, eggs, and nuts), two to three servings a day.

↪ At the very top of the food pyramid, to be used sparingly, are fats, oils, and sweets.

How many servings do you need? Almost everyone should eat at least the minimum number from each food group. What is a serving? Good question. One serving in the Grain Products Group is a slice of bread (make that whole wheat) or a bowl of cereal (three-fourths of a cup). A whole sandwich for lunch would count as two servings of grain. A cup of spaghetti for dinner counts as two servings.

A serving of fruit is any piece of fresh fruit (apple, orange, banana, for example), a half-cup of canned fruit, or three-fourths cup of fruit juice. For one serving in the vegetable category, eat a cup of leafy green lettuce-type veggies, one-half cup of cooked or chopped raw vegetables, or three-fourths cup of vegetable juice.

If you are under twenty-five years of age, you should drink three glasses of skim milk a day (or you can substitute low-fat yogurt for some of the milk). Another food in the Milk Group is cheese (one and a half ounces of natural cheese or two ounces of processed cheese).

In the Meat and Beans Group, try two ounces of lean meat, poultry, or fish. An egg, two tablespoons of peanut butter, or one-third cup of nuts count as an ounce of meat.

Some foods fit into more than one group. For example, you can count dry beans and peas as meat servings or as vegetable servings. An example given in a colorful chart published by the Education Department of the National Live Stock and Meat Board cites a large slice of sausage pizza as having ingredients in four food groups: crust (Grain Products Group), tomato sauce (Vegetable Group), cheese (Milk Group), and sausage (Meat and Beans Group). The pizza also contains a portion of your daily fat intake as well.

Put on Your Apron

You may not be the major cook in your family. And when it's PMS time, the last thing you want to do is sweat over a hot stove. But once in a while you may want to amaze your family with a well-balanced dinner, your kind of dinner. Or maybe you'd like a few recipes for easy-to-make snack foods.

Remember, your goal is to incorporate nutritious foods all month. Healthful eating will then become a pattern for you.

Many of the following sample recipes were submitted by high school and college-age women who like to cook for themselves and/or their families. Most are quick and made with readily available, PMS-fighting ingredients. You won't find any recipes with thirty or forty ingredients; most have fewer than ten things to combine. Servings may be for one person but can also be enough for two, four, or six persons. If you get into the cooking mood, you may want to invest in one or two of the many healthful-food cookbooks available at supermarkets and bookstores. Three of the many magazines that offer tips for healthful eating are: *Eating Well: The Magazine of Food & Health,*

The Nutrition Action Health Letter, and *Prevention.*
Let's start with the Grain Products Group: Cereals, Rice, Pasta, and Bread.

Grains

Nutrition experts recommend eating healthful breakfasts, and grains are a great way to start the day. If you're tired of the same old corn flakes, try adding a couple of table-spoons of dried fruits to your cereal. These days the vari-ety available is nothing short of amazing: raisins, cherries, pineapple, dates, figs, mangos, papayas. In season there are all kinds of berries, and fresh bananas are around most of the time.

If you're a hot-cereal person, you can add the same dried fruits during cooking. Also try substituting apple juice for some or all of the liquid used in cooking.

Here's a fun way to eat cereal. You could even make a few batches of Aunt Gertie's Granola for your friends.

Aunt Gertie's Granola
2 cups quick-cooking (but not instant) rolled oats
1 cup chopped, unsalted, dry-roasted, shelled peanuts
1/4 cup wheat germ
1/4 cup honey
1/4 cup apple juice
1/2 cup chopped walnuts or pecans
1 tablespoon canola oil
1/2 cup dried fruit (optional)

In a large bowl, combine oats, wheat germ, and nuts.

Combine honey, apple juice, and oil in another bowl. Add second mixture to first. Spread in a jelly-roll pan or on a cookie sheet. Bake at 300 degrees for 30 to 40 minutes or until mixture turns light brown. (Stir every 15 minutes.) Remove from oven and transfer to a cool pan. Break up chunks. Stir in dried fruit, if desired. (This addition tends to make your crunchy granola less crunchy.) Store it in containers with tight lids, or put it into plastic bags to give to your friends. They'll love it, and they'll love you too.

Couscous Cereal For One
Couscous (pronounced "koos-koos") is actually a type of pasta made from semolina flour. It comes in regular or whole-wheat varieties.

1 cup skim milk
1/4 cup raisins
2 teaspoons honey
1/3 cup whole-wheat (or regular) couscous

Heat milk, raisins, and honey in a small pan. When mixture starts to boil, pour in couscous. Cover and let stand about five minutes or until couscous is creamy. If you prefer, you can double this recipe and microwave the leftover portion the next day.

Breakfast Bulgur
If you're looking for something different for breakfast, something heartier, try cracked-wheat bulgur.

1/2 cup bulgur
1 cup water

1/4 teaspoon salt (optional)
1 teaspoon low-sugar preserves or fruit-only preserves (optional)
Skim milk (optional)

Combine bulgur and water. Bring to a boil, then reduce heat and simmer in a covered saucepan for 10 to 12 minutes until bulgur is tender and water is absorbed. Serve with low-sugar preserves and/or skim milk.

Antoinette's Easy French Toast for Two

This is another popular but simple dish you can eat anytime. Antoinette and her mother like to make it for Sunday brunch. Using "egg product," which consists of egg whites and therefore eliminates the cholesterol of egg yolks, also saves time.

1/4 cup "egg product" or two whole eggs, beaten
1/4 cup skim milk
1/4 cup orange juice
4 slices somewhat stale bread, preferably whole wheat
1 or 2 teaspoons canola oil (or enough to keep toast from sticking)

In a shallow bowl, mix eggs, milk, and juice. Place each slice of bread into mixture for five seconds. Let bread soak up the egg for five seconds on the other side. Brush a large nonstick skillet with half the oil. Cook two slices, then two more with the remaining oil. Serve with low-sugar syrup. (Like many recipes, this recipe has elements of more than one food group; in this case it's the Egg Group and the Milk Group.)

Wonderful Wheat Pancakes
1 cup whole-wheat flour
1/4 cup unbleached flour
2 tablespoons wheat germ
1 tablespoon brown sugar
1 teaspoon baking powder
1/4 teaspoon baking soda
1/4 teaspoon salt
1 egg, beaten, or 1/4 cup egg product
1 1/4 cups low-fat buttermilk
1 tablespoon canola oil

In a medium-sized bowl, combine dry ingredients. Combine liquids, except oil, in another bowl. Add liquid ingredients to dry mixture and blend. Use a small amount of the oil on a griddle or frying pan. When the grill is hot, add 1/4 cup of batter for each pancake. Turn pancakes when surface bubbles. Keep going in this manner until all of the batter is used up. Serve with fresh fruit. Makes approximately 8 pancakes.

Easy Couscous Soup for One or Two
Whether this serves one or two depends on how much you like it and also on how many other things you're having for lunch or dinner.
1 medium onion, chopped
2 medium tomatoes, chopped
2 cloves garlic, peeled and minced
1 can vegetable broth
1 cup couscous, precooked according to package directions

Salt and pepper to taste
2 tablespoons Parmesan cheese

Sauté onion, tomatoes, and garlic in a small amount of olive oil. Add vegetable broth and couscous. Bring to boiling point but don't boil. Serve with Parmesan cheese.

Wild-ish Rice

Because it is hard to grow (and mainly grows on its own in a limited area), wild rice is an expensive item. With this recipe you can fool your guests and make believe you're living on the "wild side."

1 cup regular uncooked rice (not the instant kind)
2 tablespoons margarine
1 small can (4 ounces) undrained mushrooms, sliced
1/4 teaspoon thyme
1 can consommé
1 can water (use the consomme can)
1/4 teaspoon rosemary
Nonstick vegetable spray

Spray a 9- by 13-inch baking dish with nonstick spray. Pour in all ingredients. Cover loosely with foil. Bake at 350 degrees for about an hour until liquid is absorbed and rice is tender. Stir once at about 30 minutes. Serves 4 to 6.

Cooked Brown Rice

Even better for you than white rice is brown rice (either short-grain or long-grain).

1 cup brown rice
2 cups water (If using long-grain rice, you'll need l/3

cup more water.)
1/2 teaspoon salt

Combine rice and water in a saucepan and bring water to a boil. Boil for about a minute. Reduce heat, cover pan, and simmer for about 25 to 30 minutes (or until water is gone and rice is tender).

Chickpea Sauce and Spaghetti

You don't need to add salt to this recipe because the canned chickpeas and Parmesan cheese make it salty enough.

2 15-ounce cans chickpeas, undrained
2 tablespoons vegetable oil, preferably olive
4 large cloves garlic, minced (4 teaspoons)
1 1/2 cups thinly sliced onions (1 1/2 large)
1 16-ounce can tomatoes, drained and cut up with liquid reserved
1 teaspoon rosemary, crushed
1/4 cup minced fresh parsley
Freshly ground black pepper to taste
1 pound spaghetti, cooked and drained
1/4 cup grated Parmesan cheese

In a blender, food processor, or sieve, puree 1 can of chickpeas with liquid. In a large saucepan, heat the oil and sauté the garlic and onion until garlic begins to brown. Add the tomatoes and their liquid, rosemary, chickpea puree, and the remaining can of chickpeas with liquid to the saucepan. Stirring often, heat the mixture for about 15 minutes or until it has thickened. Add parsley and pepper. Toss the hot cooked spaghetti with the sauce and sprinkle with Parmesan before serving. Serves 6.

"Szechuan" Noodles with Peanut Sauce

You only have to cook the pasta for this easy-to-prepare dish. Serve it hot or at room temperature.

12 ounces spaghetti, linguine, or similar pasta

1/3 cup hot water

1/3 cup smooth peanut butter (preferably all-natural)

2 teaspoons reduced-sodium soy sauce

2 teaspoons vinegar

2 scallions, finely chopped, divided

2 cloves garlic, very finely minced

1 teaspoon sugar

1/4 hot red pepper flakes, or more, to taste

Cook the pasta in boiling water until it's firm. Drain, set aside, and keep warm. While pasta cooks, make the sauce. In a medium bowl, blend water and peanut butter. Stir in soy sauce, vinegar, scallions, garlic, sugar, and hot pepper flakes. (Save 1 tablespoon of the scallions to put on top of the pasta when you serve it.) Combine sauce with hot spaghetti in a heated serving dish. Serves 4.

Fettucini with Fresh Herbs

This pasta recipe comes from Susan Stevens, author of *Delitefully Healthmark... Cooking for the Health of It.*

4 ounces eggless fettucini

1 clove garlic, minced

1 tablespoon olive oil

1/4 cup chopped parsley

1/3 cup chopped fresh basil

2 tomatoes, chopped

Fresh-ground black pepper

Cook pasta according to package directions, omitting salt. Drain. Sauté garlic in olive oil until golden. Add pasta, herbs, and chopped tomatoes. Season to taste with black pepper. Serves 4 as a side dish.

Pasta Salad

This recipe makes a lot (8 to 10 servings). You can either enjoy it for a couple of days or cut the recipe in half.

8 ounces corkscrew pasta

1 head romaine lettuce (or 1 pound fresh spinach)

3 ounce can black olives, sliced and drained

8 cherry tomatoes, cut in half

1 bunch green onions, chopped

8 mushrooms, sliced

1 1/2 cups frozen peas, thawed

l can (14 ounces) artichoke hearts, drained (optional)

1/4 to 1/2 cup bottled Italian dressing or 1/4 to 1/2 cup Basic Dressing #1 (end of chapter)

Cook pasta according to package directions. Pour into colander and rinse with cold water. Mix all the ingredients.

Your Basic Baked Potato

1 baking potato, scrubbed

Before baking, poke potato with a fork several times all over to prevent an explosion in the oven. Bake at 350 or 325 degrees for about an hour.

Purr-fect Potatoes

1 or 2 large potatoes of any kind, scrubbed

Olive oil or canola oil

Salt and pepper to taste

Slice potatoes into bite-sized chunks. Spread on a baking sheet and toss with a small amount of olive or canola oil. Bake at 375 degrees for 20 minutes or until potato chunks are soft in the middle. (Stir after 10 minutes.) Before serving, sprinkle with a little salt and pepper.

Two-way Potatoes (Sometimes called "Twice-Baked" Potatoes)

This is an old familiar recipe for those who like their potatoes two ways—baked and mashed.

2 large baking potatoes

Skim milk, warmed

Salt and pepper to taste

Scrub potatoes, poke with fork, and bake in a 325-degree oven for about an hour. Cut each potato in half lengthwise. Cool potato halves until you can handle them. Scoop out fleshy part of potato, leaving a "rim" of about l/4 inch. Mash potato pulp and add enough warm milk to make the potatoes creamy. Beat. Season with salt and pepper. Spoon potato mixture back into skins. Broil until slightly brown on top—about 5 minutes.

Fruits and Vegetables

Now that you've climbed to the second level of the food pyramid, greet two categories of foods that need little or

119

no preparation for eating.

Smoothies

Smoothie, citrus slush, fruit shake—these are varieties of delicious, easy-to-make fruit drinks. The following recipe will give you an idea of what you can do with some fruit and a blender. (You'll find more "smoothie" recipes in the yogurt/milk section.)

O.B. (Orange Banana) Shake
1 cup skim milk
1 ripe banana
1/4 cup frozen orange juice concentrate

Mix all in blender and drink.

Anna's Delight

This summer Anna, seventeen, has a job as a receptionist. Everyone in the office drools over the fruit she brings in a clear plastic container for lunch. Anna has mild PMS, and her healthful diet helps, and her "fruit delight" looks beautiful and tastes good. If you want to be the envy of your group, you need three or four fruits from Group 1 and at least one fruit from Group 2.

Group One: Red or green apple half (washed, sliced, and drizzled with lemon juice)

Orange or green melon balls. Watermelon is okay too, but it gets watery.

One-half banana (peeled, sliced, and drizzled with lemon juice)

A peach (washed, sliced, and drizzled with lemon juice)

A plum (washed and sliced)

Group Two: Washed grapes, strawberries, blueberries, Bing cherries, raspberries
Layer the fruits from Group One in a dish or container, then sprinkle one or two fruits from Group Two over the top. Most of the time Anna makes her concoction the night before. The lemon juice prevents discoloration.

Fruit Kabobs
If you (or someone you know) won't eat fruit, here's a way to increase your (or their) interest. Buy a package of wooden skewers, available in most supermarkets. Cut fruits into 1-inch squares. (Most fruits, except citrus fruits and melons, will need a squirt of lemon juice to prevent discoloration.) Thread on skewers alternate chunks of pineapple, cantaloupe, honeydew melon, watermelon, peaches, nectarines, apricots, bananas, and grapes. Serve before dinner as a colorful appetizer.

Rainbow Salad
4 cups mixed salad greens, washed and dried (use the greenest of greens)
1 1/2 cups cantaloupe balls
1/4 cup red onion rings, thinly sliced
1/4 cup feta or bleu cheese, crumbled
Lemon dressing
In a large salad bowl, mix all ingredients, except dressing. Just before serving, add lemon dressing. Toss salad.

Lemon dressing
1/2 cup lemon juice, freshly squeezed

1/4 cup olive oil or canola oil
1/4 teaspoon salt

My Granny's Marinated Vegetable Salad
1 cup fresh broccoli tops (florets)
1 cup carrots, sliced diagonally
1 cup cauliflowerettes
1 cup celery, sliced diagonally
1/2 cup green or red pepper strips
1/2 cup green onions, chopped
1 cup apple juice, unsweetened
1/2 cup cider vinegar
3/4 teaspoon black pepper

In a small amount of water, steam (for 3 or 4 minutes) the first four vegetables until barely tender. Cool. In a large bowl, combine steamed vegetables with peppers and onions. In a separate bowl, mix apple juice, vinegar, and pepper. Stir and cover. Refrigerate vegetables overnight.

Your Mama's Broccoli Dip
3/4 pound broccoli, cooked and liquefied in blender
1 medium onion, chopped
2 large garlic cloves, minced
1 tablespoon lemon juice
Salt and pepper to taste

Combine all ingredients and use as a dip for your homemade tortilla chips or for raw vegetables.

Aunt Nellie's Vitamin-Packed Veggies
Nellie's Veggies #1
1/2 pound fresh broccoli, washed and trimmed
1/2 pound fresh cauliflower, washed and trimmed
4 or 5 cloves garlic, peeled and chopped fine
2 tablespoons low-sodium soy sauce
2 tablespoons olive oil

Place broccoli and cauliflower on a broiler pan or cookie sheet. Mix last 3 ingredients and drizzle on veggies. Put pan on top oven rack and bake at 450 degrees until veggies are crispy and lightly browned. Watch closely; at this temperature, they can burn quickly.

Nellie's Veggies #2
This recipe uses the same vegetables but cooks them in another way, giving them a different flavor and consistency.
1/2 pound fresh broccoli, washed and trimmed
1/2 pound cauliflower, washed and trimmed
Lemon wedges
salad dressing
Steam veggies in a covered pan in a small amount of water, just barely covering them. Cook for 3 or 4 minutes until slightly tender. The broccoli should still be bright green. Serve hot or cold with lemon juice or salad dressing for dipping.

Billy Goat Gruff Greens
1/2 head romaine lettuce, washed and dried
3/4 fresh, shredded Parmesan cheese
1/4 cup regular Caesar dressing diluted with vinegar

In a large bowl, break up lettuce leaves into bite-sized pieces. Sprinkle with cheese. Just before serving, drizzle dressing over greens. Toss and eat. (If you don't mind limp lettuce, the greens will still taste good the next day.)

Erica's Colorful Cabbage
1/2 pound cabbage, shredded or sliced in fine strips
1/2 cup carrots, shredded
1/2 cup broccoli florets and stems chopped
1/2 cup cherry tomatoes, quartered
1/2 cup celery, sliced
1/2 cup fresh parsley, chopped
1/4 cup canola oil
2 tablespoons cider vinegar
1 tablespoon Dijon mustard
1/2 teaspoon salt
1/2 teaspoon pepper

In large bowl, combine cabbage, carrots, broccoli, tomatoes, and celery. Put rest of ingredients in tightly covered jar and shake well. Pour over cabbage mixture.

Baked Onion Rings
Here's a recipe for baked onion rings compliments of The American Institute for Cancer Research.
4 large onions
1 1/2 cups fine dry bread crumbs, half whole wheat, if possible
1/2 teaspoon poultry seasoning
3 tablespoons grated Parmesan cheese, optional
1 egg (for best results, don't use a substitute)

1 tablespoon water

Slice each onion about 1/4-inch thick and separate into rings. Soak the rings in cold, salted water for about 30 minutes. Drain on paper towels. Combine bread crumbs, poultry seasoning, and Parmesan cheese. In a separate bowl, mix egg and water. Beat. Dip onion rings into bread crumb mixture, into the egg mixture, then back into the crumbs. Arrange rings on a greased jelly-roll pan or cookie sheet. Cover with foil and bake in 400-degree oven for about 10 minutes. Remove foil and bake for 20 more minutes or until crispy.

Oven Stew

This stew contains meat, but it fits here in the vegetable category because it contains onion, celery, carrots, and green beans (optional). This winter recipe cooks all by itself in the oven while you warm yourself by the fireplace.

1 pound lean beef, such as bottom round steak, cut into 1/2-inch cubes
1 medium onion, chopped
4 stalks celery, sliced
3 large carrots, sliced
1/2 pound fresh green beans (optional)
1 cup tomato juice
1 tablespoon sugar
1/2 teaspoon salt
1/2 teaspoon black pepper
1/2 teaspoon basil
2 medium red potatoes cut into small pieces (just wash

them—no need to peel)

Combine all ingredients except potatoes in a 2 1/2-quart, ovenproof, covered casserole dish or Dutch oven. Bake at 325 degrees for 3 hours. Stir several times during baking. Add water, if necessary. Stir in potatoes during last hour. Serves 6.

Meat, Poultry, Fish, Dry Beans and Peas, Eggs, and Nuts

Climbing up the pyramid, you will come next to this large group, which provides many choices for the two to three servings you need each day.

Sweet-Sour London Broil

Christine's mother gave her the following adaptation of a recipe she found in a Cincinnati newspaper thirty years ago. It was contributed by the Schmitz family, who liked to entertain at outdoor barbecues.

2 large, unscored flank steaks (about 3 pounds)
Tenderizer
1/2 cup canola oil
1/4 cup white vinegar
1/4 cup white Karo syrup
1/4 cup A-1 sauce
1/4 cup catsup
3 tablespoons Worcestershire sauce
2 tablespoons Heinz 57 sauce
5 tablespoons low-sodium soy sauce
Lightly wet steaks and sprinkle on both sides with ten-

derizer. With a fork, poke tenderizer at 1/2-inch intervals into meat. Place steaks in a 9- by 13-inch glass dish. Mix together all liquid ingredients and pour over meat, turning meat once so both sides are wet with marinade. Cook over hot coals on an outdoor grill or inside on the broiler for approximately 5 minutes on each side. With a sharp knife, cut thin slices across the grain at a 45-degree angle. This version makes enough for 6 to 8 persons, but you can make half the recipe if you prefer.

Spicy Chicken
1/4 teaspoon garlic powder
2 teaspoons ground cumin
2 teaspoons chili powder
1/4 teaspoon salt
1/2 teaspoon black pepper
1 teaspoon sugar
3 tablespoons Worcestershire sauce
1 pound (approximately) boneless, skinless chicken breasts (you can also use bone-in chicken breasts and remove the skin)
Nonstick vegetable spray

In a small bowl, mix the first seven ingredients. Spray a 9 by 13-inch glass dish with non-stick spray. Place chicken pieces in dish and pour liquid mixture over them. Cover lightly with foil. Bake at 350 degrees for 40 minutes or until chicken is done.

Easy Oriental Chicken
3 tablespoons low-sodium soy sauce

2 tablespoons honey
1 teaspoon peeled, grated fresh ginger
2 cloves garlic, peeled and minced
1 pound (or slightly more) boneless chicken breasts, skinned
Nonstick vegetable spray

In a small bowl, combine first 4 ingredients. Set aside while you pound (good for discharging your feelings) the chicken to a thickness of 1/4 inch. Spray a broiler rack with nonstick vegetable spray. Grill about 3 minutes on each side. During cooking, baste with soy sauce mixture.

Buttermilk Chicken
4 chicken breasts, skinned (if you use boneless chicken, reduce cooking time)
1/2 teaspoon garlic, peeled and minced
1/4 teaspoon paprika
1 teaspoon tarragon
1/2 teaspoon salt
1/2 teaspoon pepper
1 tablespoon onion flakes, dehydrated
1 cup buttermilk
Arrange chicken in a 9- by 13-inch, ovenproof baking dish. Combine rest of ingredients and pour over chicken. Cover and bake at 325 degrees for 45 minutes; remove cover and bake for 30 more minutes.

Chicken in Currant Sauce
This recipe is very simple, delicious, and impressive. Your relatives will think you can really cook. You can.

About 1 pound boneless, skinless chicken breasts
1 medium onion, sliced
1/2 cup water
1/4 cup currant jelly or preserves
1 tablespoon Dijon-style mustard
Put all ingredients in a large skillet. Bring liquid mixture to a boil, reduce heat and simmer for 25 to 30 minutes or until done. During cooking, turn breasts at least once. Also watch carefully. If the liquid evaporates, add a little water. (This recipe is from the American Institute for Cancer Research.)

Simple Salmon (on the grill)
4 8-ounce salmon fillets
Olive or canola oil
Salt and pepper to taste
Lemon wedges

Make sure the grill is clean; brush with oil. Use medium heat. Brush fillets on both sides with oil. Sprinkle with salt and pepper. Grill for about 5 or 10 minutes on each side, depending on the thickness of the fillets. Fish is done when the center of the fillet turns light pink. (You can also use the broiler for this recipe.) Serves 4.

Marinated Garbanzos
1 can chickpeas, drained and rinsed with cold water
Basic Dressing #1 at end of this chapter, or use a bottled Italian dressing
Pour a small amount of dressing over chickpeas; marinate for several hours. Add to a green salad at serving time.

Baked Garbanzos

1 can chickpeas, drained
1 teaspoon olive oil

Toss peas with oil. Bake for an hour (stirring occasionally) at 350 degrees. Eat as a snack or use in salads. Store in refrigerator; they don't stay fresh forever. You now have in your hand a good source of fiber, B-6, iron, and magnesium. (This information is compliments of *Prevention*, November 1996.)

Ha-Ha-Hot Bean Dip

Bean dip tastes good and is good for you. There are many variations; the well-known Mideastern hummus is only one example. You can use bean dips with raw veggies, tortilla chips, or as a sandwich spread with pita bread.

1 can "chili beans"
1/2 cup picante sauce (mild, medium, or hot)

Blend beans first. Then add picante sauce and give the mixture another whirl. Good as a dip.

Mexican Bean Salad

1 l6-ounce can black beans, drained
1 cup canned corn, drained
1/2 cup Italian dressing or 1/4 cup Basic Dressing #1 (at end of chapter)
4 ounces cheddar cheese
2 fresh tomatoes, quartered
4 cups washed and dried romaine or leaf lettuce, torn into small pieces

Mix beans and corn with dressing. Marinate at least an hour. Divide lettuce onto four salad plates. Spoon corn and bean mixture over lettuce. Sprinkle cheese on top. Decorate with tomatoes.

Easy Lasagna with Beans
This recipe looks long, but it's easy to make because you don't have to cook the noodles ahead of time.
1 tablespoon canola oil
1 teaspoon garlic, peeled and minced
1 small onion, chopped
2 cups canned kidney beans, drained, rinsed, and chopped
2 cups tomato sauce
2 cups tomato puree (tomato paste)
1 teaspoon oregano
1 teaspoon basil
3/4 pound *uncooked* lasagna noodles, white or wheat
1 cup cottage cheese
1 cup soft tofu, mashed and mixed with cottage cheese
8 ounces (1 cup) part-skim Mozzarella cheese, grated
1/4 cup grated Parmesan cheese (optional)

Sauté garlic and onions in canola oil. Stir in beans. Add tomatoes and spices. Bring to a boil, reduce heat, and simmer for 10 minutes. Spread a third of the bean mixture on the bottom of a 9- by 13-inch glass dish. Layer a third of the noodles on top of the beans. On top of the noodles, put half of the cottage cheese-tofu mixture. Then add Mozzarella. Keep repeating layers until everything is used up. Cover with foil and bake at 350 degrees for an hour or until noodles are soft. Sprinkle Parmesan cheese on top.

Split Pea with Mushroom Soup

This recipe uses green or yellow split peas, which usually need soaking. If you cook the soup long enough, however, they will soften up.

1 tablespoon canola oil
1 medium onion, chopped
2 cloves garlic, peeled and minced
3/4 cup yellow or green split peas
1 cup sliced mushrooms
1 medium carrot, peeled and chopped or 10 baby carrots, cut into small pieces
4 cups low-salt chicken broth
1/2 teaspoon black pepper
Salt to taste

Rinse peas in colander. In a large saucepan, sauté onion, garlic, celery, carrots, and mushrooms until softened. Add chicken broth and split peas. Reduce heat, cover, and simmer soup for 45 minutes or until peas are soft. Stir occasionally. At this point, you can eat the soup and see all the veggies you're eating, or you can cool the soup for 10 minutes, pour the mixture into a blender, and whirl until soup is creamy. Reheat and eat. Serves 4.

Lentil Chili

Lentils are tiny flat seeds that pack a wallop of fiber. Lentils cook in 20 to 30 minutes without prior soaking.

1/2 pound lentils

5 cups water
1/2 teaspoon salt (or to taste)
1 large onion, chopped
1 bay leaf
1 clove garlic, peeled and minced
1/2 pound lean ground pork or lean ground turkey
16 ounces tomato sauce
10 ounces tomato juice
8 ounces cold water
1 or 2 tablespoons chili powder

In colander under running water, rinse lentils. Put in large covered pan with bay leaf and water. Bring lentils to a boil, reduce heat, and simmer for 30 minutes. Drain water. Brown ground pork or turkey with onion, garlic, and salt. Combine meat mixture with drained lentils. Add tomato sauce, tomato juice,water, and chili powder. Cook for 1 hour to blend flavors.

Spicy Vegetable Stew
This easy-to-make stew was adapted from a friend's "African Stew" recipe. It uses chickpeas and makes a lot, so you can freeze some if you want to.
1 large onion, chopped
1 large clove garlic, peeled and chopped
1 tablespoon canola oil
3 cups fresh spinach, chopped (or kale, or Swiss chard, if you can find it)
1/2 cup raisins
1 can (15 1/2) chickpeas, drained
1 large can (28 ounces) tomatoes, chopped or blended,

or 4 to 5 fresh tomatoes, chopped
2 yams (or 2 red-skinned potatoes), scrubbed or peeled, chopped
1/2 cup uncooked, slow-cooking rice
1/2 teaspoon black pepper
Salt to taste

Fry onion and garlic in canola oil. Add chopped spinach and sauté until limp. Add rest of ingredients, except salt. Cook for 45 minutes or until yams or potatoes are soft when pricked with a fork. Add salt to taste. (If stew gets too thick, add water or a small can of tomato juice or sauce.)

Good Eggs
2 thin slices boiled ham, Canadian bacon, or turkey bacon, chopped
3 green onions, sliced
1/4 pound sliced, fresh mushrooms sautéed with 1 teaspoon low-sodium soy sauce
1 cup egg product (or 4 eggs)
5 ounces (1 1/4 cups) cheddar cheese, shredded
1/2 cup skim milk
1/4 teaspoon black pepper
Nonstick vegetable spray

Spray nonstick vegetable oil on bottom and sides of a 8- or 9-inch casserole dish. Sauté onions with mushrooms in soy sauce for about 5 minutes. Combine this mixture with rest of ingredients in medium bowl. Pour into casserole. Bake uncovered for 35 to 40 minutes. Serves 4.

Crustless Quiche

Try this crustless quiche for breakfast, brunch, lunch, or dinner.

1 tablespoon onion, chopped
3/4 cup grated, Monterey Jack cheese or cheddar cheese
1 1/2 cup skim milk
3/4 cup egg product (or 3 eggs)
1/4 teaspoon dry mustard
1/2 teaspoon black pepper
Nonstick vegetable spray

Spray non-stick vegetable oil on bottom and sides of 8- or 9-inch glass pie pan or casserole dish. Mix quiche ingredients together. Then add any of the following vegetables or a mixture of them up to 1/2 cup: sliced mushrooms, broccoli or cauliflower (cut into small pieces), diced potatoes, sliced zucchini, red or green bell peppers. Bake at 350 degrees for about 40 minutes or until set. Serves 4.

Milk, Yogurt, and Cheese

Kathy's Quick Start

Kathy says she invented this smoothie recipe. She likes it so much, she has made it every morning for the past seven years.

1/2 cup orange juice
1/2 cup skim milk
2 tablespoons any type "instant breakfast" powder
1 frozen ripe banana or one nonfrozen banana and 2 ice cubes

135

Put all ingredients in blender and whir.

Red, White, and Blueberry Smoothie
This recipe is an adaptation of a recipe from the California Milk Advisory Board.
1 cup blueberry yogurt
1 cup sliced strawberries
1 cup skim milk
6 ice cubes
Put all ingredients in blender and blend.

"Any Fruit" Smoothie
This recipe is a variation on the one above.
1 6-ounce container of yogurt with fruit (if you want to limit your sugar, use plain yogurt)
1 cup of a "matching" fruit (for example if you use peach yogurt, add fresh, canned, or frozen peaches)
1/2 cup skim milk
Throw all into blender and blend.

Fresh Fruit Smoothie
1 ripe banana, frozen, if possible
1/2 cup fresh strawberries, peaches, or apricots
1 cup plain yogurt
1/2 cup skim milk
Blend all ingredients.

Camilla's Cheese Squares
Camilla adapted this recipe from the original "Green Chile Bites," which appeared in the Junior League of

Denver's best-selling 1978 cookbook, *Colorado Cache*. It's so easy to make that she takes it to any event that requires guests to bring a snack.

1 1/2 cups egg product (or 6 eggs)
4 cups (about 1 pound) sharp cheddar cheese, grated
1 4-ounce can mild green chiles, chopped and drained
Non-stick spray

Spray the bottom and sides of an 8- by 8-inch or 9- by 9-inch baking dish. Spread green chiles on bottom of dish. Sprinkle with grated cheese. Pour egg product over cheese and chiles. Bake at 350 degrees for about 30 minutes or until firm. Cut into squares and serve warm.

Cheese-Broccoli Soup

2 cups low-sodium chicken broth
1/4 cup onion, chopped
1 cup dry milk powder
2 1/4 cups water
1/4 cup flour
1 cup cheddar cheese, shredded
1/4 teaspoon black pepper
1 package (10 ounces) frozen, chopped broccoli, thawed

In a 2-quart saucepan, heat broth and onions. Bring broth to a boil, reduce heat, and simmer for 10 minutes. Combine dry milk and 2 cups of the water. Add to broth. Bring mixture to a boil, reduce heat, and simmer for 10 more minutes. Mix remaining 1/4 cup of water with flour until mixture is smooth. Add flour mixture to broth and stir until soup mixture thickens. Add cheese, pepper, and broccoli; stir and reheat. Serves 6.

Fats, Oils, and Sweets

Basic Dressing #1
1/2 cup olive oil
1/4 cup balsamic vinegar
1/2 teaspoon salt
1/2 teaspoon black pepper
1/2 teaspoon mustard
1 teaspoon minced garlic

Combine all ingredients in a jar with a tight-fitting cover. Shake well. Use to lightly coat salad greens. Store leftover dressing in refrigerator.

Basic Dressing #2
1/2 cup olive oil
1/4 cup lemon or lime juice
1 teaspoon minced garlic
2 tablespoons oregano
1/4 teaspoon salt
1/4 teaspoon pepper

Combine in jar. Shake and use. Store leftover dressing in refrigerator.

Pumpkin Raisin Bread
1 1/2 canned pumpkin puree
1/2 cup honey or sugar

1/2 cup melted butter
2 eggs, slightly beaten
1/2 cup raisins
1/2 cup walnuts, chopped
1 cup flour
1/2 cup fine yellow cornmeal
1/2 cup rolled oats
1 teaspoon baking powder
1/2 teaspoon ground cinnamon
1/2 teaspoon ground allspice
1/4 teaspoon ground nutmeg
1/4 teaspoon ground ginger
1/4 teaspoon ground cloves
1/2 teaspoon salt

Preheat oven to 350 degrees. In a medium-sized bowl, mix the pumpkin, honey, melted butter, and eggs. Stir in milk, raisins, and walnuts. In another bowl, mix the the dry ingredients together and make a big well in the center. Slowly pour in the pumpkin mixture and mix only until ingredients are blended. Try not to overwork the batter. Pour the batter into a well-greased 6 by 9-inch loaf pan. Bake one hour. Let cool for ten minutes before cutting.

You can find (or invent) more healthy recipes to add to those in this chapter. You might even want to get a notebook or recipe file and start your own collection.

Learning to Live with PMS

Whether you suffer from mild or severe PMS symptoms,

you've learned here that it is a manageable problem. Unlike other illnesses, PMS is difficult to diagnose. When you break a bone, there's an x-ray to show the fracture. When you cut yourself, you bleed. But PMS symptoms are internal and vague. For many sufferers, it's hard to describe their feelings and hard to find sympathy, let alone a doctor who will listen with a serious and caring ear. But it can be done. It's a matter of taking control over your PMS and doing something about it.

It's natural to want to be taken care of when dealing with any illness. If you're like most people, you want others to know how you feel—without having to tell them—and then take care of you. When you have a cold, your mom brings soup and tender-loving care. But if you have PMS, it's up to you to figure out what makes you feel good, and then do it. Or you have to patiently explain to someone how you are feeling, and even then that person might not be as helpful or understanding as you'd like. But following some of the suggestions in this book will help your symptoms and help you take control over your life. The benefits of dealing with your PMS through a healthful lifestyle, anger management, improved communication skills, and possible counseling will not only relieve your symptoms, but give you skills to improve all facets of your life.

Glossary

adhesions Abnormal scar tissue that sometimes causes body organs to "stick together."

anovulatory menstrual cycle Menstrual cycle in which the expected ovulation does not occur.

areola Circle of dark skin in the middle of the breast.

breast self-examination (BSE) Technique women use to examine their breasts for suspicious lumps.

certified nurse midwife (CNM) Nurse with specialized training (and certification) in all areas of pregnancy and birthing.

cervix The lower part of the uterus, which protrudes into the upper part of the vagina.

clitoris The female part most sensitive to sexual stimulation.

complex carbohydrates Group of foods that includes fruits, vegetables, cereals, grains, and legumes.

dysmenorrhea Painful menstruation.

embryo One of the early stages of a developing fetus.

endocrine glands Ductless glands that secrete hormones into the bloodstream.

endometriosis Condition in which tissue ordinarily lining the uterus appears in other parts of the body, such as the abdominal cavity.

endometrium The lining of the uterus.

estrogen One of two female hormones produced by the ovaries.

fallopian tubes Tubes on each side of the uterus; also called oviducts or egg tubes.

fertilization The entrance of the sperm into the egg; can be

141

done in the laboratory (in vitro fertilization) and also in a woman's body.

fibroadenomas Harmless breast lumps that tend to occur most often in women under the age of forty.

follicle An unripened egg.

follicle-stimulating hormone (FSH) A pituitary hormone that stimulates the production of follicles in the ovary and the production of estrogen.

fundus The upper area of the uterus.

genes Biologic units of heredity.

genitals The external sexual organs of men and women.

gynecology The science and specialty of diseases of the female reproductive tract.

hormones Chemical substances produced by the endocrine glands and secreted into body fluids to effect certain kinds of organ functioning.

hymen Thin membrane that covers (or partially covers) the vaginal opening.

intercourse (sexual intercourse) Sexual union involving the placement of a male penis into a female vagina.

labia majora External genitals; "large lips" on each side of the labia minora.

labia minora External genitals; "small lips" on each side of the clitoris and urethra.

laparoscope An instrument used for looking into the abdominal and other body cavities; also used for surgery.

legumes Peas and beans, such as lima beans, garbanzos, kidney beans, lentils, and navy beans.

luteal phase The second half of the menstrual cycle after the rupture of the follicle.

luteinizing hormone (LH) A pituitary hormone that stimulates the production of progesterone.

mammary glands Small glands along with their associated tubules that produce milk in the breast.

manic depression Mental condition in which periods of inappropriate "highs" alternate with disabling "lows;" sometimes called bipolar disorder.

masturbation Self-stimulation of sexual organs.

menopause The time of a woman's life when her periods stop, sometime between the ages of forty and fifty-five.

menstrual cycle A monthly cycle including the making of hormones, the thickening of the uterine lining, the shedding of the uterine lining, and menstruation (bleeding).

menstruation Female monthly bleeding sometimes called a "period."

mons (also **mons pubis** or **mons veneris**) Fleshy area over the joining of the pubic bones (pubic symphysis).

nipple The small raised area and duct at mid-breast through which breast milk passes.

nurse practitioner A nurse with extra training in various medical specialties.

orgasm The peak and release of sexual tension.

ovaries The two female organs that contain eggs (ova).

ovum Egg released by an ovary during ovulation; plural form, ova.

pelvic inflammatory disease (PID) An infection, often caused by sexually transmitted germs, that spreads from the uterus to other internal female organs.

peritoneum Abdominal cavity.

pituitary gland A small endocrine gland near the brain that secretes numerous hormones.

premenstrual syndrome (PMS) A group of physical and emotional symptoms that recur in a cyclic manner in the luteal phase of the menstrual cycle.

progesterone Female hormone produced just before ovulation.

psychiatrist Medical doctor with specialized training in mental and emotional disorders.

psychologist A person with a master's degree or Ph.D. in psychology.

psychotherapy Generally refers to "talking therapy" with a counselor of some kind.

puberty The period of rapid physical, hormonal, and emotional change that occurs in young women between the ages of ten and sixteen; puberty occurs somewhat later in young men.

pubic region In both males and females, the area at the top of and between the legs.

reproductive organs The bodily parts involved with pregnancy.

triglycerides Fats in the bloodstream.

urethra The short, thin tube extending from the bladder to the outside of the body.

uterus Hollow organ with thick walls that expands during pregnancy to accommodate the baby.

vagina The expansive "tube" through which menstrual blood flows or a baby travels to the outside; sometimes called the birth canal.

vulva The external genitals of a female.

womb Another name for the uterus.

Where to Go for Help

If you or someone you know has PMS, the following organizations may be of help. Most provide educational brochures and some will refer you to local resources.

American College of Obstetricians and Gynecologists
P.O. Box 96920
Washington, DC 20090-6920
(202) 638-5577

Center for Health Sciences
c/o Institute for the Study of Human Knowledge
P.O. Box 381069
Cambridge, MA 02238-1069
(800) 222-4745

Full Circle Women's Health
1800 30th Street
Boulder, Colorado 80301-1015
(303) 440-7100
(800) 418-4040

Institute for Mental Health Initiatives
4545 42nd Street NW
Washington, DC 20016
(202) 364-7111

National Women's Health Network
514 Tenth Street NW
Washington, DC 20004
(202) 347-1140

Office of Research Reporting
National Institute of Child Health and Human
 Development (NICHD)
NIH, Building 31, Room 2A32
9000 Rockville Pike
Bethesda, MD 20205

Planned Parenthood Federation of America
Educational Resources
810 Seventh Avenue
New York, NY 10019
(212) 541-7800

PMS Access
P.O. Box 9326
Madison, WI 53715
(800) 222-4PMS (4767)

U.S. Department of Health and Human Services
Public Health Service
National Institutes of Health
Rockville, MD 20857
(800) 421-4211

For Further Reading

Beckelman, Laurie. *Anger.* New York: Crestwood House, 1994.

Bender, Stephanie DeGraff. *PMS: Questions & Answers.* Los Angeles: The Body Press, 1989.

Berger, Gilda. *PMS: Premenstrual Syndrome*: A Guide for Young Women, 3rd ed. Alameda, CA: Hunter House, 1991.

Boston Women's Health Book Collective. *The New Our Bodies, Ourselves: A Book by and for Women,* Updated and Expanded for the 1990s. New York: Simon & Schuster, 1992.

Brody, Jane. *Jane Brody's Good Food Book: Living the High-Carbohydrate Way.* New York: W.W. Norton, 1985.

Cameron, Julia. *The Artist's Way: A Spiritual Path to Higher Creativity.* New York: G.P. Putnam's Sons, 1992.

Caudill, Margaret. *Managing Pain Before It Manages You.* New York: Guilford Press, 1995.

Dalton, Katharina, M.D. *Once a Month: The Original Premenstrual Tension Handbook,* 4th rev. ed. Claremont, CA: Hunter House, Inc., Publishers, 1990.

Davies, Jill. *Premenstrual Syndrome: Special Diet Cookbook.* Great Britain: Thorsons, 1991.

Hahn, Linaya. *PMS: Solving the Puzzle: Sixteen Causes of PMS and What to Do About It.* Evanston, IL: Chicago Spectrum Press, 1995.

Kahaner, Ellen. *Everything You Need to Know About Growing*

Up Female. rev. ed. New York: The Rosen Publishing Group, 1997.

Madaras, Lynda, with Area Madaras. *The What's Happening to My Body? Book for Girls,* rev. ed. New York: Newmarket Press, 1988.

Metcalf, C. W. and Roma Felible. *Lighten Up: Survival Skills for People Under Pressure.* Reading, MA: Addison-Wesley Publishing Company, 1992.

Peter, Laurence J., M.D. and Bill Dana. *The Laughter Prescription.* New York: Ballantine Books, 1982.

Sullivan, Jane. *The Natural Way with PMS: A Comprehensive Guide to EffectiveTreatment.* Rockport, MA: Element Books, 1996.

Index

149

rights and responsibilities as patient, 77-78, 100

S

salt and premenstrual syndrome (PMS), 36, 41-42

sanitary napkins, 17-18

sexually transmitted disease (STD), 32

sleep, adequate, 51-52

smoking, health risk of, 10

stress and premenstrual syndrome (PMS), 53-56

ways to reduce stress, 56-69

sugar and premenstrual syndrome (PMS), 36, 40-41

sunlight, benefits and dangers, 52-53

support groups, 81, 102-104

symptoms of premenstrual syndrome (PMS)

charting, 27-30, 38, 51, 68, 80

list of, 25

T

tampons, 3, 18-19

toxic shock syndrome (TSS), 19

treatments for premenstrual syndrome (PMS), 81-89

alternative therapies, 85-88

lifestyle changes, 35-73

medical, 74-86

mental counseling and therapy, 97-102

12-step program, 103

U

urethra, 10

uterus (womb), 4, 11, 12, 14, 15, 16, 30, 78, 79

V

vagina, 4, 10, 11, 12, 78

vitamin and mineral supplements for premenstrual syndrome (PMS), 81-82, 90, 107-108

vulva, 10

W

Wellness Book, The (Greiff), 67

womb, 12,

Women's Health America Group, 23